THE MATERNAL HEALTH CRISIS IN AMERICA

Barbara A. Anderson, DrPH, RN, CNM, FACNM, FAAN, professor emerita, Frontier Nursing University, Lexington, Kentucky, is the former program director of the DNP program. She was lead editor of the first and second editions of *Best Practices in Midwifery: Using the Evidence to Implement Change* (2013, 2017), lead editor of *DNP Capstone Projects: Exemplars of Excellence in Practice* (2015), and coeditor of editions two through five of *Caring for the Vulnerable: Perspectives in Nursing Theory, Research, and Practice* (2008, 2012, 2016, 2019). She has served on the board of directors of the American College of Nurse-Midwives and as the chair of the Population, Reproductive, and Sexual Health Section of the American Public Health Association. She has a long career in nursing, public health and nurse-midwifery, field-based teaching, mentorship, program planning, curriculum development, and academic administration. She is a referee for *Social Science & Medicine* and the *International Journal of Childbirth* and was recently awarded the 2018 Media Award by the American Association of Birth Centers.

Lisa R. Roberts, DrPH, RN, FNP-BC, FAANP, associate professor of nursing and director of research, Loma Linda University School of Nursing, Loma Linda, California, practices as a family nurse practitioner (FNP) in a community-based clinic focusing on primary care, prevention, and preconception care. She is coeditor of *Midwifery for Nurses in India* and an author of *Caring for the Vulnerable: Perspectives in Nursing Theory, Practice, and Research*, Fourth Edition (2016). Her research involves maternal health from a public health perspective and she has published manuscripts in the *Journal of Community Health*, *International Journal of Childbirth*, *Health Care for Women International*, *Issues in Mental Health Nursing*, and *Family & Community Health*. She has taught nurses and midwives internationally and is the former program director of the FNP program at the Loma Linda University School of Nursing.

THE MATERNAL HEALTH CRISIS IN AMERICA

Nursing Implications for Advocacy and Practice

Barbara A. Anderson, DrPH, RN, CNM, FACNM, FAAN
Lisa R. Roberts, DrPH, RN, FNP-BC, FAANP

SPRINGER PUBLISHING COMPANY

Springer Publishing Company, LLC
11 West 42nd Street
New York, NY 10036
www.springerpub.com
http://connect.springerpub.com

Acquisitions Editor: Elizabeth Nieginski
Compositor: Amnet Systems

ISBN: 978-0-8261-4072-2
ebook ISBN: 978-0-8261-4084-5
Instructor's PowerPoints: 978-0-8261-3687-9
DOI: 10.1891/9780826140845

Instructor's Materials: Qualified instructors may request supplements by emailing textbook@springerpub.com.

19 20 21 22 / 5 4 3 2 1

The author and the publisher of this Work have made every effort to use sources believed to be reliable to provide information that is accurate and compatible with the standards generally accepted at the time of publication. Because medical science is continually advancing, our knowledge base continues to expand. Therefore, as new information becomes available, changes in procedures become necessary. We recommend that the reader always consult current research and specific institutional policies before performing any clinical procedure. The author and publisher shall not be liable for any special, consequential, or exemplary damages resulting, in whole or in part, from the readers' use of, or reliance on, the information contained in this book. The publisher has no responsibility for the persistence or accuracy of URLs for external or third-party Internet websites referred to in this publication and does not guarantee that any content on such websites is, or will remain, accurate or appropriate.

Library of Congress Cataloging-in-Publication Data

Names: Anderson, Barbara A. (Barbara Alice), 1944– author. | Roberts, Lisa
  R., author.
Title: The maternal health crisis in America : nursing implications for
  advocacy and practice / Barbara A. Anderson, DrPH, RN, CNM, FACNM, FAAN,
  Lisa R. Roberts, DrPH, RN, FNP-BC, FAANP.
Description: New York, NY : Springer Publishing Company, LLC, [2019] |
  Includes bibliographical references and index.
Identifiers: LCCN 2019007219 (print) | LCCN 2019011101 (ebook) | ISBN
  9780826140845 (eBook) | ISBN 9780826140722 (print : alk. paper)
Subjects: LCSH: Maternal health services—United States. |
  Mothers—Mortality—United States.
Classification: LCC RG940 (ebook) | LCC RG940 .A53 2019 (print) | DDC
  362.198200973—dc23
LC record available at https://lccn.loc.gov/2019007219

Contact us to receive discount rates on bulk purchases.
We can also customize our books to meet your needs.
For more information please contact: sales@springerpub.com

Barbara A. Anderson: https://orcid.org/0000-0002-3240-9500
Lisa R. Roberts: https://orcid.org/0000-0003-3722-8634

Printed in the United States of America.

To Angela, Jaime, Crystal, Allison, Melissa, Emma,
Jenny, Sarah, Tony, and Susan

Their stories in this book are
composite narratives of many mothers
we have cared for as nurses.
We thank them for being our best teachers—for sharing
the face of suffering and death among mothers in America.

Where is my mama?
. . . she's gone to heaven, little one . . .

Why did she go away?
. . . poor, alone, sick in a nation swirling in wealth . . .

But why did she go away?
. . . she tried so hard to stay . . . her only thought was of you . . .

But where is my mama?

—Barbara A. Anderson

CONTENTS

CONTRIBUTORS

Barbara A. Anderson, DrPH, RN, CNM, FACNM, FAAN, Professor Emerita Frontier Nursing University, Lexington, Kentucky

Dora Barilla, DrPH, President and Founder, Partners for Better Health, Pasadena, California

Julia DeSouza, BSN, RN, Clinical Faculty—Intrapartum, Loma Linda University School of Nursing, Loma Linda, California

Lakieta Edwards, DNP, RN, CNM, WHNP-BC, Full Scope Midwifery and Women's Health, The Birth Center at Parent Child Center Community Wellness Center, Berwyn, Illinois, and West Suburban Medical Center, Oak Park, Illinois

Jennifer Foster, PhD, RN, CNM, FACNM, FAAN, Clinical Professor Emerita and Anthropologist, Lillian Carter Center for Global Health and Social Responsibility and the Nell Hodgson Woodruff School of Nursing, Emory University, Atlanta, Georgia

Eileen K. Fry-Bowers, PhD, JD, RN, CPNP-PC, Associate Professor, University of San Diego, Hahn School of Nursing and Health Science, San Diego, California

Jessica Illuzzi, MD, MS, FACOG, Associate Professor of Obstetrics, Gynecology, and Reproductive Sciences, Yale University, New Haven, Connecticut; Medical Director, Vidone Birthing Center, Yale-New Haven Hospital

Joyce M. Knestrick, PhD, RN, FNP-BC, FAANP, President, American Association of Nurse Practitioners, Austin, Texas

Nancy K. Lowe, PhD, RN, CNM, FACNM, FAAN, Professor and Chair, Division of Women, Children, and Family Health, College of Nursing, University of Colorado, Denver, Colorado; Editor, *Journal of Obstetric, Gynecologic & Neonatal Nursing (JOGNN)*

Joan MacEachen, MD, MPH, Family Practice and Obstetrics, Alaska Native Tribal Health Consortium, Kodiak, Alaska

Shafia M. Monroe, DEM, CDT, MPH, President, Shafia Monroe Consulting-Birthing CHANGE, Portland, Oregon

Lisa R. Roberts, DrPH, RN, FNP-BC, FAANP, Associate Professor of Nursing and Director of Research, Loma Linda University School of Nursing, Loma Linda, California

Susan E. Stone, DNSc, RN, CNM, FACNM, FAAN, President, American College of Nurse-Midwives; President, Frontier Nursing University, Lexington, Kentucky

Suzan Ulrich, DrPH, RN, CNM, FACNM, Robert Wood Johnson Foundation Executive Nurse Fellow, Ripley, New York

Sharon Nyree Williams, MFA, MBA, Storyteller, Executive Director, Central District Forum for Arts and Ideas, Seattle, Washington; Founder, The Mahogany Project; Winner in short film category, *Addicted*, 2009 Cannes Film Festival, Cannes, France

REVIEWERS

Jill Alliman, DNP, RN, CNM, FACNM, Project Director, Strong Start for Mothers and Newborns Initiative, American Association of Birth Centers, Perkiomenville, Pennsylvania

Eugene N. Anderson, PhD, Professor Emeritus (Anthropology), University of California at Riverside, Riverside, California

Trude A. Bennett, DrPH, MSW, MPH, Associate Professor Emerita, Gillings School of Global Public Health, University of North Carolina at Chapel Hill, Chapel Hill, North Carolina

Ann Cheney, PhD, Assistant Professor, Center for Healthy Communities, School of Medicine, University of California at Riverside, Riverside, California

Lorna Kendrick, PhD, RN, PMHCNS-BC, Professor and Director, School of Nursing, California State University San Marcos, San Marcos, California

Kathryn Ross, BS, Maternal and Child Health Extension Agent, Saving Mothers, Giving Life Project, U.S. Peace Corps, Lusaka, Zambia, Southern Africa

Adrienne D. Zertuche, MD, MPH, Obstetrician/Gynecologist, Atlanta Women's Healthcare Specialists, Atlanta, Georgia

FOREWORD

There is universal agreement that the death of a woman during pregnancy, childbirth, or the early months of new motherhood is a tragic event for the child/ children left motherless, the family, and the community. Why then, in the richest country in the world, the country that spends proportionately more money per birth on healthcare during pregnancy and birth than any other, is there a maternal mortality rate that is higher by any measure than all other high-resources countries? Why has it increased markedly since the beginning of the 21st century? This is the question that Anderson and Roberts ask us to consider and respond to in this book.

Current estimates are that two or three women in the United States die per day from pregnancy-related causes. Although there has been an upsurge in maternal mortality review committees at the state level and in state and federal legislation to fund these and other activities, the efforts have been retrospective in nature, focusing on existing care approaches and funding mechanisms. Instead, analyses are needed that begin upstream to reconsider the origins of poor maternal health and preventable maternal death. We need to develop new strategies or revitalize old ones for providing care for women during pregnancy, childbirth, and the postpartum. That begins with a comprehensive understanding of the social determinants of health and the limitations of episodic medical care to foster maternal health.

It is critical to step back from the approach of simply analyzing maternal death case by case, determining why the woman died, judging whether or not the death was potentially preventable, and determining what system, facility, provider, or individual woman factors contributed to the woman's death. Comprehensive maternal mortality reviews have much to teach us about knowledge gaps among women and their families related to pregnancy, childbirth, and its complications; gaps in facility preparedness for pregnancy-related complications and emergencies; gaps in providers' knowledge and responsiveness to signs and symptoms of these complications; and gaps in coordination of care within and among healthcare facilities. However, these lessons do not cause us to question the very structure and content of care for women during childbearing. They simply lead us to plug holes rather than reconstruct the dam that is on the verge of breaking. It is time to look upstream, to reconsider what care women need before, during, and after pregnancy to foster their own health and well-being within the context of family and community. Maternal health matters because it is the foundation of a healthy, productive, democratic, and affirming society.

In the 20th century, Americans came to expect that health and healthcare would continue to improve. The great infrastructure and medical accomplishments of the 1900s, such as access to safe water, effective treatment of infectious diseases, safe blood transfusion to treat hemorrhage, and safe anesthesia for surgery, ushered in decades of advances in medical care that created the illusion that healthcare providers can handle almost anything and stave off death until old age under most circumstances. A more realistic perspective helps us realize that such is not the case. As America entered and embraced the 21st century, disparities in health outcomes due to the multifactorial influences of poverty and racism, old and emerging infections, obesity, opioid and other addictions, and increasingly obvious gaps in access to healthcare plague our country. For the first time in over 100 years, these factors have resulted in the decline of life expectancy among Americans. The illusion that America is a country of health is just that—an illusion that is highly dependent on where you live, the color of your skin, and your economic and educational resources. Each of these issues is pertinent to maternal health in America.

Anderson and Roberts ask us to consider these issues from a combined public health, nursing, and midwifery perspective. Modern nursing was founded on the concepts of public health, case finding, and holistic care, concentrating on the family in the context of community. There was a time several decades ago in nurse-midwifery education in the United States that admission requirements included experience as a public health nurse. During the last half of the 20th century, this perspective was lost in midwifery education and diluted in nursing education. This change resulted from the need for nurses in hospitals with increasingly high-acuity patient populations; the decline in public health funding for maternal–child services; and the expansion of midwifery to include women's healthcare across the life span. Maternity care became a component of women's healthcare rather than a specialty unto itself. It became dominated by the surgical specialty of obstetrics and gynecology. The reimbursement systems became based on medical services rather than holistic, family-centered care oriented to promote maternal health, self-responsibility for health, parenting skills, and the central role of the mother in her child's health. I remember with fondness a sweatshirt worn by the first female obstetrician I ever met in the 1970s, a sweatshirt with the words "We deliver healthy families" emblazoned on the back. As a young mother myself at the time, I was heartened by this physician's concentration on the woman and her family, rather than simply "getting her delivered." I also remember the inherent rightness of my ability as a nurse to refer any woman or infant to our local public health department for nursing home follow-up after hospital discharge. I became a midwife because of my desire to care for women and their families throughout the reproductive cycle with an emphasis on health promotion and the prevention or mitigation of complications and disease.

As I look back on more than 50 years of professional life as a nurse and a midwife, this book gives me hope—hope that nurses and midwives are seeing the big picture and can be emboldened to respond to America's crisis in maternal health by direct action at all levels of healthcare policy and healthcare provision. Women matter, each mother matters, and maternal health matters. Although human history clearly teaches that healthcare utopia is beyond human capabilities, I can envision a day in America when maternal health has its rightful place as a foundation of healthcare—a day when regardless of geography, race, or economics, all women have access to family planning services; holistic, woman- and family-centered care during childbearing; and ongoing postpartum care focused on individual needs in the context of family and community. The vast majority of this care can be provided by nurses and midwives.

I would like to have the power to issue an edict that every nursing, midwifery, medical, public health, and health policy student, practitioner, and educator read this book. It is that important. This book has the potential to unite us in a common cause of improving maternal health in America through collective advocacy and action. I extend my gratitude to Barbara A. Anderson and Lisa R. Roberts for writing it. It is, of course, too late for the women who die from pregnancy-related causes today, but it is not too late for America's future mothers, their children, and their families.

Nancy K. Lowe, PhD, RN, CNM, FACNM, FAAN
Editor, *Journal of Obstetric, Gynecologic & Neonatal Nursing (JOGNN)*
Professor and Chair, Division of Women, Children, and Family Health
College of Nursing, University of Colorado, Denver, Colorado
2018 Winner, Hattie Hemschemeyer Award,
American College of Nurse Midwives

PREFACE

As maternal healthcare providers and mothers, we have experienced the joy of participating in new life. We have also faced the other side—the crippling of health and the loss of life among mothers. This book is about the crisis in maternal health in America and the high number of American mothers who are sick and dying as they give life.

Our nation has seen a sharp rise in maternal deaths in the past few decades. Estimated maternal mortality ratio is 26.4/100,000 (Global Burden of Disease 2015 Maternal Mortality Collaborators, 2015). The United States ranks 46th among 183 countries and has the highest maternal death rate among all high-resource nations. Maternal morbidity and "near misses," unplanned events that did not but easily could have resulted in death, are also very high (Amnesty International, 2011; Central Intelligence Agency, 2018). Contrary to popular misconception, African American mothers or mothers in poverty are not the only ones who die or bear the burden of illness, although unquestionably they are disproportionally affected. Our nation is struggling with an emerging epidemic for which we do not have clear answers.

In this work, we challenge the current approach that embeds maternal care into child health and women's health, defining the mother as *vessel* for child health and *cause* for preterm and ill babies. We address mothers as distinct, not defined in terms of "the other." We present the current risks to maternal health and life, a crisis in the landscape of America.

This book is a reservoir of critical questions about maternal health in America—the social determinants, structural and systemic forces, the culture of healthcare, the public health safety net, and national media attention to the issue. We seek to engage nursing, public health and other healthcare students, educators, providers, and advocates in conversation about solutions to this national dilemma. We present critical thinking exercises encouraging readers to create road maps for practice and advocacy. We include a PowerPoint presentation for face-to-face and online learning. All narratives in this book are composite stories and any resemblance to the living or the dead is coincidental.

The editors are grateful to the contributors, reviewers, and the many thoughtful persons who have engaged in discussion and offered suggestions. We wish to acknowledge Springer Publishing Company and its outstanding staff: Margaret Zuccarini, publisher emerita, Elizabeth Nieginski, publisher, Rachel Landes, associate acquisitions editor, and Hannah Hicks, assistant editor. Thank you for your ever-present guidance and encouragement. We also acknowledge Billie Anne Gebb, MSLS, director of Library Services, Frontier Nursing University, who has an uncanny ability to find references and sources, no matter how obscure. We thank Bellies to Babies founder and CEO, Corrinna Edwards, CBE, PFS, for sharing the photographs of the Safe Motherhood quilts. We acknowledge the technical skills of Andrew Youmans, MS, CNM, in preparing camera-ready photographs.

To our colleagues—nurses, public health professionals, physicians, midwives, nurse practitioners, advocates for maternal health—and all those who pour out their life energies promoting the health of our mothers: We share with you the vision that American mothers may survive and thrive.

Qualified instructors may obtain access to ancillary PowerPoints by emailing textbook@springerpub.com.

Barbara A. Anderson
Lisa R. Roberts

REFERENCES

Amnesty International. (2011). *Deadly deliver: The maternal health crisis in America, one-year update, Spring 2011*. Retrieved from https://www.amnestyusa.org/reports/deadly -delivery-the-maternal-health-care-crisis-in-the-usa

Central Intelligence Agency. (2018, January 1). *The world factbook*. Retrieved from https:// www.cia.gov/library/publications/the-world-factbook/rankorder/2223rank.html

Global Burden of Disease 2015 Maternal Mortality Collaborators. (2015). Global, regional, and national levels of maternal mortality, 1990–2015: A systematic analysis for the Global Burden of Disease Study 2015. *Lancet, 388*(10053), 1775–1812. doi:10.1016/ S0140-6736(16)31470-2

MATERNAL HEALTH IN AMERICA

Mortality, Morbidity, and Near Misses

BARBARA A. ANDERSON | LISA R. ROBERTS

OBJECTIVES

At the end of this chapter, the reader will be able to:

1. Describe emerging trends of maternal mortality and severe maternal morbidity (SMM) in the United States in relation to the global maternal health data.

2. Discuss the issues in reporting accurate rates of maternal mortality and SMM in the United States.

3. Identify the leading causes in maternal mortality and SMM in the United States.

GLOBAL MONITORING OF MATERNAL MORTALITY

The World Health Organization (WHO) is the global reservoir of information on maternal mortality across the world. It ranks maternal mortality in 183 reporting nations using a standardized definition, the "maternal mortality ratio." There are 193 nations in the world but 183 report to WHO with this data. WHO defines maternal death as "the death of a woman while pregnant or within 42 days of termination of pregnancy, irrespective of the duration and site of the pregnancy, from any cause related to or aggravated by the pregnancy or its management but not from accidental or incidental causes" (WHO, n.d., para. 2).

The United States has seen a sharp rise in maternal deaths in the past few decades, estimated at an increase of 27% between 2000 and 2014 (MacDorman & Declercq, 2018). The Global Burden of Disease Study (GBD, 2015) estimates the maternal mortality ratio of 26.4 deaths per 100,000 live births compared to the "pregnancy-related mortality ratio" of 17.3 deaths per 100,000 live births used by the Centers for Disease Control and Prevention (CDC, n.d.-a). The differences in these measurements are discussed in this chapter. The United States now ranks 47th of 184 nations. It is the country with the highest maternal death rate among high-resource nations and the rate is higher than some low-resource nations (Central Intelligence Agency [CIA], 2019). National Public Radio (NPR) has spotlighted maternal deaths in its ongoing series, *Lost Mothers: Maternal Mortality in the U.S.* (Martin & Montage, 2017). Various organizations estimate the annual number of deaths among American mothers at:

- 1,200 (Agrawal, 2015)
- 1,063 (GBD, 2015)
- 700 (CDC, 2017)

The number, whatever it may be, is small compared to the loss of women globally due to maternal mortality (302,950 annually or 830 per day; WHO, United Nations International Children's Emergency Fund, United Nations Population Fund, World Bank Group, & United Nations Population Division, 2015). The United States spends more money on maternity care than any other nation in the world. Yet it lags significantly behind other high-resource nations in maternal health outcomes (Amnesty International, 2011; Chen, Chauhan, & Blackwell, 2018; Miller & Belizán, 2015). Maternal mortality decreased 44% globally between 1990 and 2015, as the Millennium Development Goals (MDGs) and the Sustainable Development Goals (SDGs) had been implemented by the United Nations (UN) and participating governments around the world (MacDorman & Declercq, 2018). Most high-resource nations implemented these UN strategies and experienced a 48% decline in maternal mortality during this period (MacDorman & Declercq, 2018). Unlike other nations, the United States has not implemented these strategies, nor has the nation adopted the 1987 WHO Safe Motherhood Initiative as national policy. The United States has not met the global MDGs or SDGs or the national goals as set forth in the Healthy People 2010 Initiative (National Center for Health Statistics [NCHS], n.d.; UN, n.d.; UN Development Programme, n.d.).

TRACKING MATERNAL MORTALITY IN THE UNITED STATES

There are widely differing statistics about the number of mothers in America who have died, experienced SMM, or barely escaped death, "near misses." Dedicated public health and clinical professionals have struggled to make sense of shifting numbers and calculation systems. Has mortality and morbidity actually increased? What are the causes? Is the escalating trend a statistical artifact? How are we analyzing the numbers? How consistently are we collecting, counting, reviewing, and reporting data across the nation? How do our data methodologies compare with international data? These are some of the key questions plaguing public health epidemiologists and healthcare clinicians. One point on which all agree is that the landscape for childbearing has changed and we are facing a crisis in maternal health in America.

The United States does not have systematic data collection or consistent analysis of maternal deaths and many states lack maternal mortality review boards (Agrawal, 2015). Only about 50% of states have maternal review boards (Clark & Belfort, 2017). The U.S. data do not compare well across states. Widely different time frames are used to define maternal mortality (MacDorman, Declercq, Cabral, & Morton, 2016). Comparison with international figures is also difficult. The U.S. coding system for maternal mortality changed in 2000 with the addition of a single question on death certificates for females, querying whether the death was a maternal death according to the WHO definition (MacDorman & Declercq, 2018; MacDorman et al., 2016).

Not all states have adopted this question. Changes in death certificate forms have been slow and inconsistent. As of 2015, three states had not adopted the new system: Alabama, West Virginia, and California. California's maternal death rate had already declined, due to statewide attention to the issue, and currently is the best in the nation (MacDorman & Declercq, 2018).

Collecting Maternal Mortality Data

There are three means of surveillance that the United States uses to collect maternal mortality data. These systems are:

- National Vital Statistics System (NVSS)
- Pregnancy Mortality Surveillance System (PMSS)
- State-Level Maternal Mortality Review Committees (St. Pierre, Zaharatos, Goodman, & Callaghan, 2018)

National Vital Statistics System

The NVSS is the national database. The NCHS, a part of the CDC, collects and disseminates data from NVSS within the nation and internationally. The data are extrapolated from death certificates with ICD-10 codes. The standard WHO definition for maternal mortality is used (NCHS, 2017). However, for over a decade now, the data in the United States have suffered from underreporting and overreporting due to deficient verification of maternal status, inconsistent coding, and inadequate surveillance and analysis. States have latitude to define and how they report maternal mortality, resulting in inconsistency. The NCHS has not published an official maternal mortality figure since 2007 (Creanga, 2018; MacDorman & Declercq, 2018; MacDorman et al., 2016; Molina & Pace, 2017).

Pregnancy Mortality Surveillance System

In addition, the CDC, using a different measure, the "pregnancy-related mortality ratio," identifies the number of maternal deaths as well as causes of death, for example, hemorrhage or eclampsia. This measure links maternal death certificates with fetal death certificates and birth certificates to obtain additional data. It also extends the time frame for capturing maternal deaths. The CDC-designated data management system, the PMSS, uses the following definition for pregnancy-related mortality ratio: the number of pregnancy-related deaths per 100,000 live births from the duration of the pregnancy through the 1st year postpartum (CDC, n.d.-a).

The data include *any* cause of death caused by pregnancy complications, a cascade of events initiated by pregnancy, or exacerbation of a fatal condition due to the physiology of pregnancy (CDC, n.d.-a; Creanga et al., 2014). The pregnancy-related mortality ratio does not include injuries or *incidental causes of death* (homicide, suicide, drug-related deaths, and accidents; CDC, n.d.-a; MacDorman & Declercq, 2018; Molina & Pace, 2018). In 2013, the CDC (2017) published the average national pregnancy-related mortality ratio as 17.3 while simultaneously identifying racial differences in mortality:

- 12.7 deaths per 100,000 live births for White women

- 43.5 deaths per 100,000 live births for Black women

- 14.4 deaths per 100,000 live births for women of other ethnicities (CDC, n.d.-a)

These differences and other social determinants of mortality and morbidity will be discussed later in the book.

State-Level Maternal Mortality Review Committees

A key function of PMSS is tracking trends and outcomes in collaboration with state-level maternal mortality review committees. However, not all states have maternal mortality review committees (CDC Foundation, 2016). Regardless of data collection differences, the numbers show that more mothers are dying, and for different reasons from 20 years ago (Amnesty International, 2011; CDC, n.d.-a, 2017; Creanga, Syverson, Seed, & Callaghan, 2017; Shaw et al., 2016). The nation faces a crisis in maternal deaths and severe illness.

THE CAUSES OF MATERNAL MORTALITY

Increasingly, pregnant women in the United States have chronic diseases, for example, hypertension, diabetes, obesity, and heart disease, as well as older age of childbearing (age 35–44). The upward trend in maternal comorbidities correlates with the increased mortality and morbidity (CDC, 2017; Creanga, 2018; Creanga et al., 2015, 2017; Fisher, Kim, Sharma, Rochat, & Morrow, 2013; Florio, Daming, & Grodzinsky, 2018; Metcalfe, Wick, & Ronksley, 2018; Vaught et al., 2018). As of 2012, 44.1% of pregnant women had at least one comorbidity (Florio et al., 2018; Metcalfe et al., 2018). In the United States, up to 50% to 60% of maternal deaths are preventable. Maternal deaths are rooted not only in pathology but also in

TABLE 1.1 Causes of Maternal Deaths, 2011–2013

PREGNANCY-RELATED CAUSE OF DEATH	% OF DEATHS
Cardiovascular diseases	15.5
Noncardiovascular diseases	14.5
Infection or sepsis	12.7
Hemorrhage	11.4
Cardiomyopathy	11.0
Thrombotic pulmonary embolism	9.2
Hypertensive disorders of pregnancy	7.4
Cerebrovascular accidents	6.6
Unknown cause of death	6.1
Amniotic fluid embolism	5.5
Anesthesia complications	0.2

SOURCE: Centers for Disease Control and Prevention. (n.d.-a). Pregnancy Mortality Surveillance System. Retrieved from https://www.cdc.gov/reproductivehealth/maternalinfanthealth/pmss.html

contributing factors: patients' lack of knowledge, provider misdiagnosis or ineffective treatment, or a fragmented healthcare system (Amnesty International, 2011; Building U.S. Capacity to Review and Prevent Maternal Deaths, 2018; Creanga et al., 2015; MacDorman & Declercq, 2018; Zuckerwise & Lipkind, 2017).

As Table 1.1 demonstrates, maternal mortality in the United States is closely tied to diseases of the heart and vascular system (CDC, n.d.-a). The mortality from these diseases in pregnancy has been increasing (CDC, n.d.-a; Creanga et al., 2015, 2017; Smilowitz et al., 2018). The rate of acute myocardial infarction (AMI) has risen significantly between 2002 and 2014 with over 50% of the deaths occurring in the postpartum (Smilowitz et al., 2018). Cardiovascular diseases and cardiomyopathy represent 26.5% of pregnancy-related deaths, but chronic illnesses, hypertensive disorders, and cerebrovascular accidents impact pathology of the heart and vascular system (see Table 1.1). Cumulatively, the impact on maternal mortality is enormous.

Peripartum Cardiomyopathy

Peripartum cardiomyopathy, an initial onset of heart failure during pregnancy or within the first 5 months postpartum (Hilfiker-Kleiner, Haghikia, Nonhoff, & Bauersachs, 2015), is a serious and understudied public health problem. There are enormous differences in incidence, outcomes, mortality, and need for cardiac transplant between African American women and non-African American women

(Gentry et al., 2010; Irizarry et al., 2017; Kolte et al., 2014). Key risk factors, chronic hypertension, pregnancy-induced hypertension, and preeclampsia, can often be managed with adequate care (Bello, Rendon, & Arany, 2013; Bibbins-Domingo et al., 2009; Hilfiker-Kleiner et al., 2015). Racial disparity in adequacy of care is discussed in the next chapter.

Noncardiovascular Diseases

Noncardiovascular chronic diseases, for example, type 1 and type 2 diabetes, kidney disease, cancer, and autoimmune diseases such as systemic lupus erythematosus (SLE), are also killers in pregnancy (Building U.S. Capacity, 2018; CDC, n.d.-a). SLE is an example of a devastating, noncardiovascular disease that contributes to preeclampsia, eclampsia, kidney failure, and maternal death (Ling, Lawson, & Scheven, 2018). Obesity, especially morbid obesity, is an overarching problem exacerbating most chronic conditions and can contribute to mortality through increased risk for cardiovascular disease, postpartum hemorrhage, and puerperal infection (Aughinbaugh & Carlson, 2017; Fisher et al., 2013).

Infections and Sepsis

Infections can be lethal in pregnant and puerperal woman, as Semmelweis demonstrated, when he introduced handwashing as a lifesaving measure (Markel, 2015). Lethal infections during childbearing can result in puerperal sepsis, septic abortion, pyelonephritis/urosepsis, or virulent soft tissue infections. Chlamydia and gonorrhea are caused by pathogens that can create life-threatening sepsis (Gravett et al., 2012). HIV/AIDS and hepatitis, two prevalent infections, may *contribute* to mortality (Al-Ostad, Kezouh, Spence, & Abenhaim, 2015). A death from influenza, however, can be *pregnancy related* (Callaghan, Creanga, & Jamieson, 2015). Sepsis is a major cause of mortality (CDC, n.d.-a). Death from septic abortion is particularly tragic since abortion is a legal procedure in the United States. The occurrence of sepsis in pregnancy doubled between 2001 and 2010 along with a rise in sepsis-related maternal death (Acosta et al., 2013; Al-Ostad et al., 2015; Creanga et al., 2017; Oud & Watkins, 2015). Sepsis concurrent with renal disease, chronic liver disease, heart failure, and HIV/AIDS leads to the highest sepsis-related maternal mortality (Al-Ostad et al., 2015).

The risk for peripartum stroke during delivery is increased in the presence of an infection, according to a recent study (Miller et al., 2018). Any infection during delivery increases the risk of peripartum stroke (adjusted odds ratio 1.74), but especially genitourinary infections (adjusted odds ratio 2.56) and sepsis (adjusted odds ratio 10.4). The confidence level was 95% for all findings. The participants in this case-control cohort study (n = 455 cases/1,365 controls) had a mean age of 29.8 years (Miller et al., 2018).

Catastrophic Events

Fatal hemorrhage, hypertensive complications (e.g., eclampsia), and anesthesia-related problems have declined (Creanga et al., 2017). Embolism is less preventable, although astute care in the peripartum by health professionals can quickly identify it. The birth experience of the tennis champion Serena Williams exemplifies the need for patients to be their own advocates when healthcare professionals do not actively listen (Scutti, 2018).

With enhanced protocols and initiatives, eclampsia and deadly placenta previa, abruption, and accreta are less likely to be catastrophic. Anesthesia-related deaths have also decreased, although there is concern over the continuing high rate of medical intervention, induction, and cesarean section, which are associated with increased mortality (Amnesty International, 2011; Callaghan, Creanga, & Kuklina, 2012).

The Medicalization of Childbirth

Physiologic birth is the ideal and is being promoted by numerous professional and lay organizations. Nonetheless, the rates of cesarean section and induction remain very high, well above the levels recommended by the WHO.

Cesarean Section

Nationally, the average cesarean delivery rate (including both medically necessary and maternal request) is approximately 33%, while WHO's recommendation is 10% to 15% (Lagrew et al., 2018). States with rates over 33% have higher risks of maternal mortality from surgical complications, infections, pneumonia, cardiac arrest, and venous thrombosis (Amnesty International, 2011; Schuiling & Slager, 2017; Shamshirsaz & Dildy, 2018). Primary cesarean birth accounts for 50% of the sharp increase, posing the need to avoid primary cesareans unless absolutely necessary (Barber et al., 2011).

Cesarean birth increases the risk for future impaired fertility and complications or mortality from placenta previa or accreta (Lagrew et al., 2018; Schuiling & Slager, 2017). In 2010, the National Institutes of Health (NIH) held a conference on vaginal birth after cesarean (VBAC), concluding that VBAC is a reasonable, safe option for many women. To enable most women to select this option, barriers in the healthcare system need to be addressed (Leslie, 2017; NIH, 2010).

Induction

Induction of labor has increased in tandem with increase in cesarean birth, although the overall rates have slightly declined (Kozhimannil, Macheras, & Lorch, 2014; Schuiling & Slager, 2017). The national trend to induce labor prior to full term, defined as before 39 weeks' gestation, has resulted in concerns about preterm birth, forced labor due to unripe cervix, epidural placement, increase in cesarean birth rate, and postpartum hemorrhage (Kozhimannil et al., 2014; Saccone & Berghella, 2015; Snowden et al., 2016). The data on birth outcomes with induction are mixed.

Mental Health

Deaths due to mental illness are a strongly emerging trend (Building U.S. Capacity, 2018). Intimate partner violence during childbearing, depression, suicide, homicide, and drug abuse (especially opioid overdose) are looming concerns on the horizon of maternal deaths (Building U.S. Capacity, 2018).

TRACKING MATERNAL MORBIDITY IN THE UNITED STATES

SMM is much more prevalent than maternal death. Assuming 700 maternal deaths per year, the number is small in comparison to the estimated 50,000 to 60,000 women affected by life-threatening, unexpected outcomes related to birth, that is, SMM (CDC, n.d.-a, n.d.-b; Callaghan et al., 2012; Chen et al., 2018; Howell, Egorova, Balbierz, Zeitlin, & Hebert, 2016). Many of these unexpected outcomes are near misses, in which the mother barely escapes death during pregnancy, the intrapartal period or within 42 days of postpartum (Amnesty International, 2011; Chen et al., 2018). The SMM rate is calculated by comparing hospitalized birthing women who develop severe complications to a base of 10,000 hospital admissions of birthing women, that is, delivery hospitalizations (CDC, n.d.-b). For example, in 2014, the rate for all causes of SMM was 144 birthing women/10,000 delivery hospitalizations (CDC, n.d.-b). As a sentinel indicator of maternal mortality, SMM is increasing in incidence (Creanga et al., 2014; Lazariu, Nguyen, McNutt, Jeffrey, & Kacica, 2017).

Entering pregnancy with comorbidities and subsequent SMM coincide with rising maternal mortality (Agrawal, 2015; CDC, 2017; Creanga et al., 2015, 2017; Creanga, 2018; Fisher et al., 2013; Florio et al., 2018; Metcalfe et al., 2018). As with maternal mortality, SMM is largely preventable (Agostino, Wilson, & Byfield, 2016; CDC, 2017).

Tracking SMM in the United States suffers from lack of systematic and continuous data collection, just like maternal mortality (Agrawal, 2015; Creanga et al., 2014). Data on SMM are collected using the following methods:

- Disease-specific condition
- Specified intervention
- Organ-system dysfunction criteria (Creanga et al., 2014)

SMM Coded by Disease-Specific Conditions

This method mirrors the pregnancy-related mortality ratio. It identifies the cause of SMM by disease-specific condition, such as hemorrhage or infection.

Unlike mortality data, which identify the cause of death (a one-time event), SMM frequently presents as a multicausal and shifting picture. This method of data collection may not adequately assess the level of acuity, the extent of lifesaving intervention required, or the time frame for recovery. The data collection is often inconsistent with the widely different documentation in hospital records. In addition, there could be a number of variable case scenarios around a single diagnosis, for example, hemorrhage, which exemplifies the need for maternal morbidity review panels as well as maternal mortality review panels.

For instance, a 39-year-old obese mother with gestational diabetes experienced a hemorrhage after cesarean section with subsequent wound dehiscence and infection. This woman had a moderate postpartum hemorrhage, receiving one unit of blood; her gestational diabetes was resolving; and the dehiscence of the transverse cesarean incision was healing. However, she had a fever and inflamed margins of the wound. The situation was unexpected by her provider since the woman had maintained glucose control and weight management during the pregnancy. This situation could have led to death, but she survived and was discharged with her healthy infant, antibiotics, careful instructions on wound care, and teleconference follow-up. Is this a SMM? It might or might not be coded as SMM, depending upon how the data are collected.

Conversely, this woman could be a brittle type 1 diabetic with a large postpartum hemorrhage, dehiscence of an emergency vertical cesarean incision, staphylococcus infection in the wound, a raging fever with impeding septicemia, and oliguria. During her pregnancy, she had worked closely with her provider to maintain glucose control and weight management. When she entered the hospital in labor, she and her provider both anticipated a high-risk, but carefully managed, physiologic birth. A cascade of unexpected events occurred during her labor, including fetal distress. Yet, she survived and was eventually discharged, facing a long convalescence. Using disease-specific condition coding does not allow for differences in complex situations, multiple and shifting diagnoses, or clear indicators of the degree of SMM. It makes comparison of SMM data difficult and inconsistent.

Severe Maternal Mortality Coded by Specified Intervention

A second method of data collection is identifying the SMM rate per 10,000 delivery hospitalizations by high-acuity interventions rather than by disease-specific condition (CDC, n.d.-b). The most common intervention for SMM is blood transfusion, followed by hysterectomy and breathing support by mechanical ventilation or temporary tracheostomy. Using this method, the *overall rate* of SMM intervention reflects morbidity based upon the above interventions. The data are also segmented by intervention with and without transfusion, by hysterectomy intervention, and by breathing assistance. These three interventions are heroic, lifesaving measures and provide a good estimate of both acuity and extent of SMM.

The data are captured by the National Inpatient Sample (NIS), which is an extensive database sponsored by the U.S. government's Agency for Healthcare Research and Quality (AHRQ; Healthcare Cost and Utilization Project, 2018).

The data from 1993 to 2014, examined from this perspective, have revealed a 200% overall increased rate of SMM (49.5 to 144/10,000 delivery hospitalizations). This change reflects mostly a fivefold increase in the use of blood transfusion. Excluding blood transfusion, the SMM rate in the same time period increased from 28.6 to 35/10,000 delivery hospitalizations (CDC, n.d.-b). Although rarer than blood transfusions for managing SMM, hysterectomy, which effectively limits further fertility to use of a surrogate, increased by 55% (6.9 to 10.7/10,000) and the use of breathing assistance increased by 93% (4.1 to 7.9/10,000) in this time period (CDC, n.d.-b).

SMM Coded by Organ-System Dysfunction Criteria

Of the three methods, coding by organ-system dysfunction criteria shows the most potential in establishing standardization of criteria (Callaghan et al., 2012; Creanga et al., 2014). Two working groups from the WHO have proposed this approach in capturing SSM and near misses (Firoz et al., 2013; Say, Souza, Pattinson, & WHO Working Group on Maternal Mortality and Morbidity Classifications, 2009). The CDC uses ICD-10 diagnosis and procedure codes linked to hospital discharge records to establish 18 key indicators of SMM related to organ-system dysfunction (Callaghan et al., 2012; CDC, n.d.-b) in addition to the high-acuity interventions described earlier (see Box 1.1).

BOX 1.1

KEY INDICATORS OF SEVERE MATERNAL MORBIDITY

Acute myocardial infarction
Aneurysm
Acute renal failure
Adult respiratory distress syndrome
Amniotic fluid embolism
Cardiac arrest/ventricular fibrillation
Conversion of cardiac rhythm
Disseminated intravascular coagulation
Eclampsia
Heart failure/arrest during surgery or procedure
Puerperal cerebrovascular disorders
Pulmonary edema/acute heart failure
Severe anesthesia complications
Sepsis

(continued)

(*continued*)

Shock

Sickle cell disease with crisis

Air and thrombotic embolism

Other major interventions (blood transfusion, hysterectomy, temporary tracheostomy, and ventilation)

SOURCE: Centers for Disease Control and Prevention. (n.d.-b). Severe maternal morbidity in the United States. Retrieved from https://www.cdc.gov/reproductivehealth/maternalinfanthealth/smm/severe-morbidity-ICD.htm

LEADING CAUSES OF SMM

SMM has been increasing along with the rise in cesarean births, increased comorbidities, preexisting health conditions, and more mothers at advanced age for pregnancy (Campbell et al., 2013; Callaghan et al, 2012; Fisher et al., 2013; Lisonkova et al., 2017; Martin, Hamilton, Osterman, Driscoll, & Matthews 2017; Small et al., 2012). Cardiac events, such as AMI, are a leading cause of SMM (Building U.S. Capacity, 2018; Callaghan et al., 2012; Small et al., 2012; Smilowitz et al., 2018). In the CDC study of nine states, 95% of the resulting deaths after SMM occurred in relation to:

- Cardiac arrest/ventricular fibrillation
- Conversion of cardiac rhythm
- Mechanical ventilation (Building U.S. Capacity, 2018)

The major causes of SMM are identified as the key indicators in the organ-system dysfunction criteria, for example, acute renal failure, shock, respiratory distress, and aneurysms (Callaghan et al., 2012).

One large outcome study (n = 685,228 deliveries) examined SMM at delivery and subsequent hospital encounters at 6 weeks and 1 year after delivery. The study participants all experienced SMM but had no history of preexisting chronic conditions. The SMM rate was 99/10,000 among this assumed healthy population without preexisting chronic conditions. In the two time frames of the study, 2.8% of these women were readmitted to the hospital and 1% had short-term observational stays in the hospital (95% confidence interval; Harvey et al., 2017). This study exemplifies the extent of SMM, even among women without preexisting conditions. Chronic health issues, risky behaviors, older age of childbearing, and depression, combined with racism, poverty, geographical isolation, inadequate numbers of healthcare providers, lack of available maternal healthcare, and a weak public health safety net, undermine the well-being of mothers in America. In sum, the maternal health crisis is a perfect storm, an epidemic of lost mothers, reflecting the lack of national political will and entrenched structural and systemic forces that impact family development and the cohesion of a multicultural nation. In the following chapter, we discuss these social determinants of maternal health.

SUMMARY

Approximately 50% to 60% of maternal deaths in the United States are preventable, rooted not only in pathology but in contributing factors: patients' lack of knowledge and comorbidities, provider misdiagnosis or ineffective treatment, and healthcare system factors. Additionally, flawed data collection systems for maternal morbidity and mortality limit reliable national statistics for accurate tracking and comparison with other nations.

WHAT IF

This section poses critical questions about the crippling of health and the loss of life among America's mothers. It is an opportunity to think creatively about solutions. Answers are deliberately not provided. The solutions to this national epidemic lie in interdisciplinary, imaginative conversation and problem solving. The authors invite the readers to consider these questions and add additional ones.

MATERNAL HEALTH

How would accurate, consistent reporting of maternal mortality and SMM contribute to the ability to address these issues?

How likely will the trajectory in maternal mortality and morbidity continue given the current healthcare system in America?

Discuss the top indicators of maternal mortality and morbidity. What can be done to modify these indicators and how likely would this be to change maternal health?

Can the trends in maternal mortality and morbidity be reversed without increasing high healthcare expenditure? If so, what needs to be done?

REFERENCES

Acosta, C., Knight, M., Lee, H., Kurinczuk, J., Gould, J., & Lyndon, A. (2013). The continuum of maternal sepsis severity: Incidence and risk factors in a population-based cohort study. *PLosOne, 3*(8), e67175. doi:10.1371/journal.pone.0067175

Agostino, M., Wilson, B., & Byfield, R. (2016). Identifying potentially preventable elements in severe adverse maternal events. *Journal of Obstetric, Gynecologic & Neonatal Nursing, 45*(6), 865–869. doi:10.1016/j.jogn.2015.12.016

Agrawal, P. (2015). Maternal mortality and morbidity in the United States of America. *Bulletin of the World Health Organization, 93*(3), 133–208. doi:10.2471/BLT.14.148627

Al-Ostad, G., Kezouh, A., Spence, A., & Abenhaim, H. (2015). Incidence and risk factors of sepsis mortality in labor, delivery and after birth: Population-based study in the

USA. *Journal of Obstetrics and Gynaecology Research, 41*(8), 1201–1206. doi:10.1111/jog.12710

Amnesty International. (2011). *Deadly delivery: The maternal health care crisis in the USA: One-year update.* New York, NY: Author. Retrieved from https://cdn2.sph.harvard.edu/wp-content/uploads/sites/32/2017/06/deadlydeliveryoneyear.pdf

Aughinbaugh, L., & Carlson, N. (2017). Evidence-based midwifery care for obese childbearing women. In B. A. Anderson, J. P. Rooks, & R. Barroso (Eds.), *Best practices in midwifery: Using the evidence to implement change* (2nd ed., pp. 109–129). New York, NY: Springer Publishing Company.

Barber E., Lundsberg, L., Belanger, K., Pettker, C., Funai, E., & Illuzzi, J. (2011). Indications contributing to the increasing cesarean delivery rate. *Obstetrics & Gynecology, 118*(1), 29–38. doi:10.1097/AOG.0b013e31821e5f65

Bello, N., Rendon, I., & Arany, Z. (2013). The relationship between pre-eclampsia and peripartum cardiomyopathy: A systematic review and meta-analysis. *Journal of the American College of Cardiology, 62*(18), 1715–1723. doi:10.1016/j.jacc.2013.08.717

Bibbins-Domingo, K., Pletcher, M. J., Lin, F., Vittinghoff, E., Gardin, J. M., Arynchyn, A., . . . Hulley, S. B. (2009). Racial differences in incident heart failure among young adults. *New England Journal of Medicine, 360*(12), 1179–1190. doi:10.1056/NEJMoa0807265

Building U.S. Capacity to Review and Prevent Maternal Deaths. (2018). *Report from nine MMRCs.* Retrieved from http://reviewtoaction.org/Report_from_Nine_MMRCs

Callaghan, W., Creanga, A., & Jamieson, D. (2015). Pregnancy-related mortality due to influenza in the United States during the 2009–2010 pandemic. *Obstetrics & Gynecology, 126*, 486–490. doi:10.1097/AOG.0000000000000996

Callaghan, W., Creanga, A., & Kuklina, E. (2012). Severe maternal morbidity among delivery and postpartum hospitalizations in the United States. *Obstetrics & Gynecology, 120*(5), 1029–1036. doi:10.1097/AOG.0b013e31826d60c5

Campbell, K., Savitz, D., Werner, E., Pettker, C., Goffman, D., Chazotte, C., & Lipkind, H. (2017). Maternal morbidity and risk of death at delivery hospitalization. *Obstetrics & Gynecology, 122*(3), 627–633. doi:10.1097/AOG.0b013e3182a06f4e

Centers for Disease Control and Prevention. (n.d.-a). Pregnancy Mortality Surveillance System. Retrieved from https://www.cdc.gov/reproductivehealth/maternalinfanthealth/pmss.html

Centers for Disease Control and Prevention. (n.d.-b). Severe maternal morbidity in the United States. Retrieved from https://www.cdc.gov/reproductivehealth/maternalinfanthealth/severematernalmorbidity.html

Centers for Disease Control and Prevention. (2017). *Maternal health: Advancing the health of mothers in the 21st century.* Retrieved from https://www.cdc.gov/chronicdisease/resources/publications/aag/pdf/2016/aag-maternal-health.pdf

Centers for Disease Control and Prevention Foundation. (2016). CDC Foundation partnership to help reduce maternal mortality in the United States. Retrieved from https://www.cdcfoundation.org/pr/2016/cdc-foundation-partnership-help-reduce-maternal-mortality-united-states

Central Intelligence Agency. (2019). The world factbook. Retrieved from https://www.cia.gov/library/publications/the-world-factbook/rankorder/2223rank.html

Chen, H., Chauhan, S., & Blackwell, S. (2018). Severe maternal morbidity and hospital cost among hospitalized deliveries in the United States. *American Journal of Perinatology, 35*(13), 1287–1296. doi:10.1055/s-0038-1649481

Clark, S., & Belfort, M. (2017). The case for a national maternal mortality review committee. *Obstetrics & Gynecology, 130*(1), 198–202. doi:10.1097/AOG.0000000000002062

Creanga, A. (2018). Maternal mortality in the United States: A review of contemporary data and their limitations. *Clinical Obstetrics & Gynecology, 61*(2), 296–306. doi:10.1097/GRF.0000000000000362

Creanga, A., Berg, C., Ko, J., Farr, S., Tong, V., Bruce, C., & Callaghan, W. (2014). Maternal mortality and morbidity in the United States: Where are we now? *Journal of Women's Health, 23*(1), 3–9. doi:10.1089/jwh.2013.4617

Creanga, A., Berg, C., Syverson, C., Seed, K., Bruce, F., & Callaghan, W. (2015). Pregnancy-related mortality in the United States, 2006–2010. *Obstetrics & Gynecology, 125*(1), 5–12. doi:10.1097/AOG.0000000000000564

Creanga, A., Syverson, C., Seed, K., & Callaghan, W. (2017). Pregnancy-related mortality in the United States, 2011–2013. *Obstetrics & Gynecology, 130*(2), 366–373. doi:10.1097/AOG.0000000000002114

Firoz, T., Chou, D., von Dadelszen, P., Agrawai, P., Vanderkruik, R., Tuncalp, O., . . . The Maternal Morbidity Working Group. (2013). Measuring maternal health: Focus on maternal morbidity. *Bulletin of the World Health Organization, 91*(10), 794–796. doi:10.2471/BLT.13.117564

Fisher, S., Kim, S., Sharma, A., Rochat, R., & Morrow, R. (2013). Is obesity still increasing among pregnant women? Prepregnancy obesity trends in 20 states, 2003–2009. *Preventive Medicine, 56*(6), 372–378. doi:10.1016/j.ypmed.2013.02.015

Florio, K., Daming, T., & Grodzinsky, A. (2018). Poorly understood maternal risks of pregnancy in women with heart disease. *Circulation, 137*(8), 766–768. doi:10.1161/CIRCULATIONAHA.117.031889

Gentry, M. B., Dias, J. K., Luis, A., Patel, R., Thornton, J., & Reed, G. L. (2010). African-American women have a higher risk for developing peripartum cardiomyopathy. *Journal of the American College of Cardiology, 55*(7), 654–659. doi:10.1016/j.jacc.2009.09.043

Global Burden of Disease Study Maternal Mortality Collaborators. (2015). Global, regional and national levels of maternal mortality, 1990–2015: A systematic analysis for the Global Burden of Disease Study 2015. *Lancet, 2016*(388), 1775–1812. doi:10.1016/S0140-6736(16)31470-2

Gravett, C., Gravett, M., Martin, E., Bernson, J., Khan, S., Boyle, D., . . . Steele, M. (2012). Serious and life-threatening pregnancy-related infections: Opportunities to reduce the global burden. *PLoS Medicine, 9*(10), e1001324. doi:10.1371/journal.pmed.1001324

Harvey, E., Ahmed, S., Manning, S., Diop, H., Argani, C., & Strobino, D. (2017). Severe maternal morbidity at delivery and risk of hospital encounters within 6 weeks and 1 year postpartum. *Journal of Women's Health 27*(2), 140–147. doi:10.1089/jwh .2017.6437

Healthcare Cost and Utilization Project. (2018). Overview of the National (Nationwide) Inpatient Sample (NIS). Retrieved from https://www.hcup-us.ahrq.gov/nisoverview.jsp

Hilfiker-Kleiner, D., Haghikia, A., Nonhoff, J., & Bauersachs, J. (2015). Peripartum cardiomyopathy: Current management and future perspectives. *European Heart Journal, 36*(18), 1090–1097. doi:10.1093/eurheartj/ehv009

Howell, E., Egorova, N., Balbierz, A., Zeitlin, J., & Hebert, P. (2016). Black-White differences in severe maternal morbidity and site of care. *American Journal of Obstetrics & Gynecology, 214*(1), 122, e121–122, e127. doi:10.1016/j.ajog.2015.08.019

Irizarry, O., Levine, L., Lewey, J., Boyer, T., Riis, V., Elovitz, M., & Arany, Z. (2017). Comparison of clinical characteristics and outcomes of peripartum cardiomyopathy between African American and non–African American women. *JAMA Cardiology, 2*(11), 1256–1260. doi:10.1001/jamacardio.2017.3574

Kolte, D., Khera, S., Aronow, W., Palaniswamy, C., Mujib, M., Ahn, C., . . . Fonarow, G. (2014). Temporal trends in incidence and outcomes of peripartum cardiomyopathy in the United States: A nationwide population-based study. *Journal of the American Heart Association, 3*(3), e001056. doi:10.1161/JAHA.114.001056

Kozhimannil, K., Macheras, M., & Lorch, S. (2014). Trends in childbirth before 39 weeks' gestation without medical indication. *Medical Care, 52*, 649–657. doi:10.1097/ MLR.0000000000000153

Lagrew, D. C., Low, L. K., Brennan, R., Corry, M. , Edmonds, J., Gilpin, B. G., . . . Jaffer, S. (2018). National partnership for maternal safety: Consensus bundle on safe reduction of primary cesarean births—supporting intended vaginal births. *Obstetrics & Gynecology, 131*(3), 503–513. doi:10.1097/AOG.0000000000002471

Lazariu, V., Nguyen, T., McNutt, L., Jeffrey, J., & Kacica, M. (2017). Severe maternal morbidity: A population-based study of an expanded measure and associated factors. *PLoS One, 12*(8), e0182343. doi:10.1371/journal.pone.0182343

Leslie, M. (2017). Vaginal birth after cesarean: Emotion and reason. In B. A. Anderson, J. P. Rooks, & R. Barroso (Eds.), *Best practices in midwifery: Using the evidence to implement change* (2nd ed., pp. 369–391). New York, NY: Springer Publishing Company.

Ling, N., Lawson, E., & Scheven, E. (2018). Adverse pregnancy outcomes in adolescents and young women with systemic lupus erythematosus: A national estimate. *Pediatric Rheumatology, 16*(26), 1–6. doi:10.1186/s12969-018-0242-0

Lisonkova, S., Potts, J., Muraca, G., Razaz, N., Sabr, Y., Chan, W., & Kramer, M. (2017). Maternal age and severe maternal morbidity: A population-based retrospective cohort study. *PLosMed, 14*(5), e1002307. doi:10.1371/journal.pmed.1002307

MacDorman, M., & Declercq, E. (2018). The failure of the United States maternal mortality reporting and its impact on women's lives. *Birth, 45*, 105–108. doi:10.1111/ birt.12333

MacDorman M., Declercq E., Cabral H., & Morton C. (2016). Recent increases in the U.S. maternal mortality rate—disentangling trends from measurement issues. *Obstetrics & Gynecology, 128*, 447–455. doi:10.1097/AOG.0000000000001556

Markel, H. (2015). In 1850, Ignaz Semmelweis saved lives with three words: Wash your hands. Retrieved from https://www.pbs.org/newshour/health/ignaz-semmelweis -doctor-prescribed-hand-washing

Martin, J., Hamilton, B., Osterman, M., Driscoll, A., & Matthews, T. (2017). Births: Final data for 2015. *National Vital Statistics Reports, 66*(1), 1–89. Retrieved from https:// www.cdc.gov/nchs/data/nvsr/nvsr66/nvsr66_01.pdf

Martin, N., & Montage, R. (2017). U.S. has the worst rate of maternal deaths in the developed world. *National Public Radio.* Retrieved from https://www.npr.org/2017/ 05/12/528098789/u-s-has-the-worst-rate-of-maternal-deaths-in-the-developed -world

Metcalfe, A., Wick, J., & Ronksley, P. (2018). Racial disparities in comorbidity and severe maternal morbidity/mortality in the United States: An analysis of temporal trends. *Acta Obstetricia et Gynecologica Scandinavica, 97*(1), 89–96. doi:10.1111/aogs.13245

Miller, S., & Belizán, J. (2015). The true cost of maternal death: Individual tragedy impacts family, community and nations. *Reproductive health, 12*(1), 56. doi:10.1186/s12978 -015-0046-3

Miller, E., Gallo, M., Kulick, E., Friedman, A., Elkind, M., & Boehme, A. (2018). Infections and risk of peripartum stroke during delivery admissions. *Stroke*, 2018(49), 1129– 1134. doi:10.1161/STROKEAHA.118.020628

Molina, R., & Pace, L. (2017). A renewed focus on maternal health in the United States. *New England Journal of Medicine, 2017*(377), 587–588. doi:10.1056/NEJMc1715957

Molina, R., & Pace, L. (2018). Correspondence: Maternal health in the United States. *New England Journal of Medicine, 2018*(378), 1705–1707. doi: 10.1056/NEJMp1709473

National Center for Health Statistics. (n.d.). Healthy People 2010. Retrieved from https:// www.cdc.gov/nchs/healthy_people/hp2010.htm

National Center for Health Statistics (2017). *Instructions for classifying the underlying cause of death, 2017.* National Center for Health Statistics instruction manual. Hyattsville, MD. Retrieved from https://www.cdc.gov/nchs/data/dvs/2a_2017.pdf

National Institutes of Health. (2010). *NIH consensus development conference statement: Vaginal birth after Cesarean: New insights.* Retrieved from http://consensus.nih.gov/ 2010/images/vbac/vbac_statement.pdf

Oud, L., & Watkins, P. (2015). Evolving trends in the epidemiology, resource utilization, and outcomes of pregnancy-associated severe sepsis: A population-based cohort study. *Journal of Clinical Medical Research, 7*(6), 400–416. doi:10.14740/jocmr2118w

Saccone, G., & Berghella, V. (2015). Induction of labor at full term in uncomplicated singleton gestations: A systematic review and metanalysis of randomized controlled trials. *American Journal of Obstetrics & Gynecology, 213*(5), 629–636. doi:10.1016/j .ajog.2015.04.004

Say, L., Souza, J., Pattinson, R., & WHO Working Group on Maternal Mortality and Morbidity Classifications. (2009). Maternal near miss—towards a standard tool for monitoring quality of maternal health care. *Best Practice & Research Clinical Obstetrics & Gynaecology, 23*(3), 287–296. doi:10.1016/j.bpobgyn.2009.01.007

Schuiling, K., & Slager, J. (2017). The limits of choice: Elective induction and cesarean delivery on maternal request. Evidence-based midwifery care for obese childbearing women. In B. A. Anderson, J. P. Rooks, & R. Barroso (Eds.), *Best Practices in midwifery: Using the evidence to implement change* (2nd ed.; pp. 393–407). New York, NY: Springer Publishing Company.

Scutti, S. (2018). After Serena Williams gave birth, "everything went bad." CNN. Retrieved from https://www.cnn.com/2018/01/10/health/serena-williams-birth-c-section-olympia -bn/index.html

Shamshirsaz, A., & Dildy, G. (2018). Reducing maternal mortality and severe maternal morbidity: The role of critical care. *Clinical obstetrics & gynecology, 61* (2), 359–371. doi:10.1097/GRF.0000000000000370

Shaw, D., Guise, J., Shah, N., Gemzell-Danielsson, K., Joseph, K., Levy, B., . . . Main, E. (2016). Drivers of maternity care in high-income countries: Can health systems support woman-centered care? *Lancet, 388*(10057), 2282–2295. doi:10.1016/S0140 -6736(16)31527-6

Small, M., James, A., Kershaw, T., Thames, B., Gunatilake, R., & Brown, H. (2012). Near-miss maternal mortality: Cardiac dysfunction as the principal cause of obstetric intensive care unit admissions. *Obstetrics & Gynecology, 119*(2 Pt 2), 250–255. doi:10.1097/ AOG.0b013e31824265c7

Smilowitz, N., Gupta, N., Guo, Y., Zhong, J., Weinberg, C., . . . Banglalore, S. (2018). Acute myocardial infraction during pregnancy and the puerperium in the United States. Retrieved from https://www.mayoclinicproceedings.org/article/S0025-6196 (18)30356-2/fulltext

Snowden, J., Muoto, I., Darney, B., Quigley, M., Tomlinson, M., Neilsen, D., . . . Caughey, A. (2016). Oregon's hard-stop policy limiting elective early-term deliveries: Association with obstetric procedure use and health outcomes. *Obstetrics & Gynecology, 128*(6), 1389–1396. doi:10.1097/AOG.0000000000001737

St. Pierre, A., Zaharatos, J., Goodman, D., & Callaghan, W. (2018). Challenges and opportunities in identifying, reviewing, and preventing maternal deaths. *Obstetrics & Gynecology, 131*(1), 138–142. doi:10.1097/AOG.0000000000002417

United Nations. (n.d.). We can end poverty: Millennium development goals and beyond 2015: Home page. Retrieved from http://www.un.org/millenniumgoals

United Nations Development Programme. (n.d.). Sustainable development goals. Retrieved from https://www.undp.org/content/dam/undp/library/corporate/brochure/SDGs _Booklet_Web_En.pdf

Vaught, A., Kovell, L., Szymanski, L., Mayer, S., Seifert, S., Vaidya, D., . . . Argani, C. (2018). Acute cardiac effects of severe pre-eclampsia. *Journal of the American College of Cardiology, 77*(1), 1–11. doi:10.1016/j.jacc.2018.04.048

World Health Organization. (n.d.). Maternal mortality ratio. Retrieved from http://www .who.int/healthinfo/statistics/indmaternalmortality/en

World Health Organization, United Nations International Children's Emergency Fund, United Nations Population Fund, World Bank Group, & United Nations Population Division (2015). *Trends in maternal mortality: 1990 to 2015: Estimates by WHO, UNICEF, UNFPA, World Bank Group and the United Nations Population Division.* Geneva, Switzerland: World Health Organization. Retrieved from http://www.who .int/reproductivehealth/publications/monitoring/maternal-mortality-2015/en

Zuckerwise, L. C., & Lipkind, H. S. (2017). Maternal early warning systems—towards reducing preventable maternal mortality and severe maternal morbidity through improved clinical surveillance and responsiveness. *Seminars in Perinatology, 41*(3), 161–165. doi:10.1053/j.semperi.2017.03.005

THE SOCIAL ENVIRONMENT

Determinants of the Maternal Health Crisis

BARBARA A. ANDERSON | LISA R. ROBERTS

At the end of this chapter, the reader will be able to:

1. Discuss the sociocultural, economic, and geographical factors that impact maternal mortality and severe maternal morbidity in the United States.

2. Describe the social environment for childbearing as it contributes to the maternal health crisis in the United States.

3. Identify emerging social determinants of the maternal health crisis in the United States.

THE SOCIAL DETERMINANTS OF MATERNAL HEALTH

Globally, poor maternal health aligns with the social determinants of health (United Nations Population Fund [UNFPA], 2012; World Health Organization [WHO], 2017). In the United States, maternal health reflects these social determinants in an environment characterized by increasing economic, geographical, cultural, and racial polarization. The United States has failed to ensure a safety net that includes all mothers (Sufrin, 2017; United Nations Human Rights Council [UNHRC], 2018). Poverty, geographical isolation, cultural and racial discrimination, neglect of mental health, and exposure to violence undermine the health of many American mothers (Building U.S. Capacity to Review and Prevent Maternal Deaths, 2018).

The Health Impact Pyramid is a model that examines the potential impact of interventions on health outcomes. At the base of the pyramid are the social determinants of health requiring political will and community-based action. At the

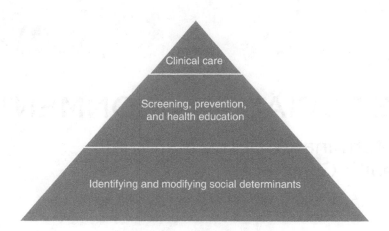

FIGURE 2.1 Maternal health pyramid of intervention.

SOURCE: Created using data from Centers for Disease Control and Prevention. (2013). *Selecting effective interventions*. Retrieved from https://www.cdc.gov/globalhealth/healthprotection/fetp/training_modules/7/selecting-interventions_ppt_final_09252013.pdf

peak are direct clinical care and information (Frieden, 2010). Maternal mortality and severe morbidity can be reduced at each level of intervention (see Figure 2.1).

Potentially, the greatest impact could occur by intervention at the base of the pyramid, modifying the social determinants that undermine maternal health (Building U.S. Capacity, 2018). It is estimated that 60% of mortality in the United States could be prevented by intervention at this level (Braveman & Gottlieb, 2014).

POVERTY

The U.S. Census Bureau estimates that 14% of Americans live in poverty (Fox, 2017). Poverty colors every aspect of a person's life. In an interlinking fashion, poverty creates unrelenting pressures for survival, necessitating harsh choices. Maternal mortality is higher among women of all races who live in poverty (Amnesty International, 2011). Some of the life stresses experienced by childbearing women in poverty are described in the following sections (see Figure 2.2).

Inadequate Housing and Transportation

Housing, or the lack of it, is frequently an overriding concern of a mother in poverty. The availability of safe, hygienic conditions for her family and herself may take precedence over other basic needs, including food. The safety of the immediate neighborhood environment, including routes to schools and employment, may be a continual stress. Having no access to readily available, safe transportation, especially at nighttime, creates safety concerns and worries about handling child care and family emergencies. Even if a poor mother has access to a car, she may not have enough money for gasoline or car repairs.

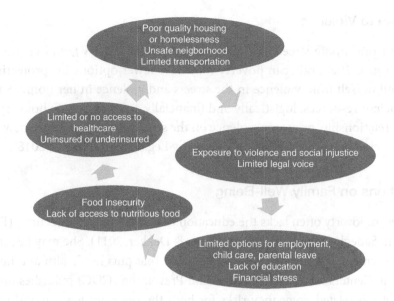

FIGURE 2.2 Interlinking elements of maternal poverty.

Sophie's Ashes

Angela was expecting her fourth child, sure this time that she would finally have a little girl after three boys. When Medicaid was finally approved, she registered at the community-based midwifery clinic but had difficulty with keeping appointments. She lacked private transportation and the local bus route was both expensive and unreliable. After two failed appointments, she arrived at the clinic without an appointment and asked to see me. I (BA) was her midwife. She stated she was bleeding. It was too late to save the pregnancy. Angela confided she could not come to the other appointments, even though she was cramping, because she had no money for the bus ticket. Angela lost her baby, returning later with a little vial of ashes. Handing them to me, she said, "Here is a little bottle with some of Sophie's ashes. I know you cared." Perhaps little Sophie could have been saved with earlier prenatal care, but Angela lost her baby for lack of a bus ticket.

Food Insecurity

Many poor families in America lack access to nutritious, fresh food, especially in inner urban and rural areas. Available foods, often from fast-food chains, may be high in calories and low in nutrients. These foods contribute to obesity and gestational diabetes (UNHRC, 2018). Beyond limited availability to food is no food at all. Poor families may have empty cupboards, as I have observed many times while practicing public health nursing. Having enough food on the table can be a major stressor for poor families (Natamba et al., 2017; Vance, 2016). Limited access to adequate nutritious food is part of the cycle of poor maternal outcomes.

Exposure to Violence

Violence from unsafe streets, intimate partner violence (IPV), and crime affects all Americans. The mother in poverty may have fewer options for protecting her family and herself from violence in the streets and violence in her home. She may lack sufficient resources, logistically and financially, to procure safe housing, leave a violent relationship, or escape violence on the streets. Legal assistance may not be readily accessible even with services offered by Legal Aid (UNHRC, 2018).

Restrictions on Family Well-Being

A mother in poverty often lacks the education to achieve financial security (Egerter, Braveman, Sadegh-Nobari, Grossman-Kahn, & Dekker, 2011). She may be forced to seek employment at a strenuous, low-paying job that puts her health and her baby at risk. The Centers for Disease Control and Prevention (CDC) publishes information about job-related pregnancy risks for both the pregnant woman and her employer (CDC, n.d.). The urgency of family financial need and limited job security in low-paying, hourly employment can override the woman's concern about safety.

When the baby arrives, the cost of child care may become a central issue. The mother's workplace may or may not offer paid leave benefits after childbirth, in spite of national efforts to legislate family leave policies. The United States does not compare with other developed nations (Neckerman, 2017). Most developed countries offer liberal family leave policies often up to a year after the birth (Neckerman, 2017). The family finances can become critical, forcing the woman to return to work before she has adequate time to recuperate. The stress of a short maternity leave, as well as the stress and cost associated with adequate child care, may impact the mother's mental health (Chatterji & Markowitz, 2012; Plotka & Busch-Rossnagel, 2018).

Barriers to Healthcare

A woman in poverty may face many barriers in obtaining care (Agostino, Wilson, & Byfield, 2016; Bryant, Worjoloh, Caughey, & Washington, 2010; Howell, Egorova, Balbierz, Zeitlin, & Hebert, 2016). A formidable barrier for the mother in poverty is the conflict of employment hours with clinic appointments. The mother may not be able to risk job security or income from an hourly wage.

Another obstacle can be health insurance status. The Affordable Care Act (ACA) has increased access for primary healthcare to manage chronic conditions prior to pregnancy (Markus, Andres, West, Garro, & Pellegrini, 2013). At the time of this writing, however, the ACA is threatened with being dismantled. In November 2018, there were 14 states that had rejected Medicaid expansion (FAMILIESUSA, 2018). Many women who do not qualify for Medicaid are unable to afford private insurance.

Delayed entry to prenatal care is generally because of lack of insurance, obtaining and waiting for Medicaid coverage approval, or finding a provider who will accept Medicaid (Health Resources and Services Administration [HRSA], 2015). In settings where Medicaid is not supported politically, the process of obtaining Medicaid for pregnancy care can be humiliating and an invasion of privacy (Bridges, 2017).

Women who are uninsured at the time of conception are more likely to have untreated, chronic health conditions (Building U.S. Capacity, 2018; Howell et al., 2016). Ironically, women who have chronic conditions would benefit most from early prenatal care. Uninsured pregnant women in the United States have a fourfold increased risk for pregnancy-related complications (Howell et al., 2016; HRSA, 2015) and a fourfold increase in maternal mortality (Agrawal, 2015). Women in poverty face multiple stresses and unrelenting pressures for survival. Healthcare may become a low priority, even if access is available (Tilden, Cox, Moore, & Naylor, 2018). Poverty dictates draconian choices.

GEOGRAPHY
Childbearing in Rural America

Contrary to the stereotype of rural women as robust from healthful, outdoor living, women in rural areas are often poor, obese, suffering from chronic illnesses, uninsured, and at long distances from healthcare (UNHRC, 2018). Education, employment opportunities, and transportation are limited (UNHRC, 2018). Access to services is often dependent upon unreliable vehicles and inadequate funds for gasoline. Rural women are primarily non-Hispanic Whites or American Indian and Alaska Natives (AIANs), representing 24% of American women living in 75% of the vast landmass of the nation (U.S. Department of Agriculture Economic Research Service, 2018). Rural demography is changing with influx of Hispanics and Asian Americans (U.S. Department of Agriculture Economic Research Service, updated 2019; U.S. Department of Health and Human Services, HRSA, & Maternal and Child Health Bureau, 2011). Rural women often have limited to no prenatal care, increasing the risk for severe maternal morbidity (American College of Obstetricians and Gynecologists [ACOG] Committee on Health Care for Underserved Women, 2014; Lazariu, Nguyen, McNutt, Jeffrey, & Kacica, 2017) and twice the risk for maternal mortality (Amnesty International, 2011; Bice-Wigington, Simmons, & Huddleston-Casas, 2015).

The Geography of Maternal Death

Location is critical when it comes to maternal mortality. Maternal mortality correlates with poverty and geography. Access to prenatal and intrapartal care, maternal healthcare providers, and Level 3 referral hospital care are some of the variables. Comparing state statistics, there is as much as a tenfold difference in maternal mortality. Table 2.1 extrapolates data from the CDC National Vital Statistics System us-

TABLE 2.1 Ranking of Selected States From Low to High Maternal Mortality Using the Standard Definition*

STATE	RANKING	# OF DEATHS/100,000 LIVE BIRTHS	REGION OF NATION
California	1	4.5	West
Massachusetts	2	6.1	Northeast
Nevada	3	6.2	West
Indiana	46	41.4	Midwest
Louisiana	47	44.8	South
Georgia	48	46.2	South

*Lowest maternal mortality is ranked #1 and highest maternal mortality is ranked #48 with two states not reporting (Alaska and Vermont).

SOURCE: CDC National Vital Statistics System, 2018. Retrieved from https://www.americashealthrankings.org/explore/health-of-women-and-children/measure/maternal_mortality/state/ALL

ing the standard definition of maternal mortality per 100,000 live births (see Table 2.1). According to this analysis, Georgia currently has the highest maternal mortality. It is worth noting that published figures fluctuate and another recent analysis by *USA Today* of CDC data slightly differed from the figures in Table 2.1, identifying Lousiana as the state with the highest mortality (Ungar, 2018).

Texas has been described in the media as the state with the highest maternal mortality. In fact, it currently ranks #43 at 34.2 maternal deaths/100,000 live births (CDC, 2018). The issue in Texas has been a rapid rise in maternal deaths, doubling between 2010 and 2014. In 2011, the Texas State Legislature cut two thirds of the budget for state-level reproductive health services, forcing 80 clinics to shut down and effectively eliminating access to care for many women (Redden, 2016). In addition, Texas (not unlike the nation as a whole) has had maternal mortality data inconsistencies. In 2016, Texas issued a comprehensive report, revised in 2019, analyzing the multiple factors contributing to the rise in maternal mortality, including the data analysis issues (Maternal Mortality and Morbidity Task Force & Texas Department of State Health Services, 2019).

Access to Maternal Healthcare in Rural America

Key to inaccessible healthcare is the lack of healthcare providers in rural facilities (Hung, Kozhimannil, Casey, Henning-Smith, & Prasad, 2016; Kozhimannil, Henning-Smith, Hung, Casey, & Prasad, 2016). Up to 40% of counties in the United States lack even one qualified maternity care provider (obstetrician, midwife, or family care physician; ACOG Committee on Health Care for Underserved Women,

2014). The result has been widespread closure of community-based and critical access hospitals providing maternity care services (Hung, Kozhimannil, Casey, & Moscovice, 2016). The workforce issue, however, is restricted not just by geography. Factors driving the critical shortage of maternity care providers across the nation are examined later in this book.

Justin Needed a Ride

Crystal, gravida 6, para 2, was a 35-year-old non-Hispanic White, living with her partner and their two young sons in an isolated, rural community. Her partner was currently out of work. She rarely kept her prenatal clinic appointments, 1 hour away. Her partner stated they did not have money for gasoline. Social services had made many attempts to help this family with transportation and other support services. I (BA) was the public health nurse assigned to visit her weekly since she was not keeping regular appointments at the clinic and had a history of pregnancy loss.

Crystal was not sure why she had lost the previous pregnancies. With this pregnancy, she had moderately elevated blood pressure and a prepregnancy body mass index (BMI) of 38. At each visit I monitored her blood pressure, urine, the heart rate and growth of the fetus, and observed for edema. Now at 34 weeks, her blood pressure was significantly higher, she complained of a headache and epigastric pain, and she had facial and ankle edema. The fetal heart was 150 and regular. I advised Crystal to go to the emergency room immediately and I notified the clinic doctor and the emergency room. I also offered to call an ambulance. Crystal's partner refused saying they had no money for an ambulance and he would take her to the emergency room, a 1-hour drive. Crystal agreed with her partner. I told them I would meet them at the emergency room.

Four hours later Crystal had not arrived at the emergency room. As the family had no telephone, I called social services who stated they would visit the family the next day. I had a bad feeling about the situation and drove back to the home. Neighbors, who were caring for the children, told me that Crystal and her partner had quarreled. He wanted to watch a football game on television before leaving for the emergency room. They told me that the couple had just now left for the emergency room and that Crystal was feeling very ill.

I returned to the emergency room where Crystal had been admitted, hemorrhaging with a placental abruption. She tested positive for cocaine. The baby was dead, and she had an emergency hysterectomy and multiple blood transfusions and was admitted to the ICU.

Later in the step-down recovery area, I visited Crystal. She was grieving and wanted to hold her lost baby. I obtained permission from the hospital to bring the baby from the morgue, dressed the little boy in a hand-knitted outfit, and brought him to his mother. Crystal held him closely, calling him Justin, and telling him she loved him. Justin died as a result of many interlinking social factors, including

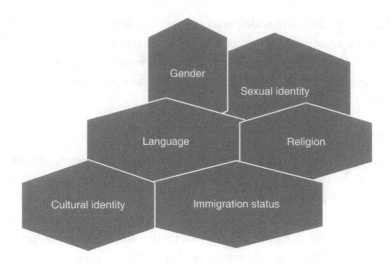

FIGURE 2.3 The many faces of maternity care.

geographical isolation. Crystal did not die but suffered life-altering morbidity and loss of fertility.

A MULTICULTURAL NATION

American mothers represent the many faces of a multicultural nation. Maternity healthcare providers need to be nimble as they interact with mothers and their families from many different backgrounds. In any patient–provider encounter, multiple facets of multiculturism may be operating on both sides. America needs maternity care providers from all of these backgrounds and providers who can transcend and relate to mothers from multiple backgrounds (see Figure 2.3).

Mothers and Providers in a Multicultural Society

In a multicultural society, each person brings a mosaic of experience. In any one clinic day, the following scenarios could be present, each one necessitating sensitivity to protecting maternal health. Each of these scenarios is offered as an opportunity for critical thinking and discussion:

- A Turkish-speaking immigrant woman wondering if anyone will understand her

- An undocumented woman terrified that her provider may betray her to immigration authorities

- A gay male obstetrician informs his female-to-male transgender male patient with an intact uterus that he has a positive pregnancy test

- A Muslim woman and her husband who will see only a female nurse-midwife

- An Ethiopian immigrant woman with genital cutting reticent to see an American family physician who she fears will criticize this practice

- A young nulliparous Asian American obstetrician caring for a 45-year-old woman who has just undergone her third round of failed assisted reproductive technology

- An African American woman, fearing discrimination and racism, tells her Latina provider that she desires to have a Black provider

- A Navajo patient desiring a nurse-midwife who will incorporate Navajo traditional rituals into her birth experience

- A family physician with a history of childhood sexual abuse experiences flashbacks while caring for a pregnant adolescent who was raped and is now pregnant

Selected Examples of Barriers Facing Mothers in a Multicultural Nation
Culture

Barriers to prenatal care are high for AIAN women. The Indian Health Service (IHS) has struggled with severe underfunding and AIAN pregnant women have high rates of late entry or no prenatal care (Building U.S. Capacity, 2018). The maternal mortality among AIAN is almost as high as African Americans at 38.8/100,000 live births (CDC, 2018).

Language

Translation can be an issue. For reasons of privacy, family members are not allowed to translate for a patient. Moreover, there may be information essential about a woman's reproductive health that a woman may not wish her family to know, particularly if translation is conducted by her child. In some healthcare environments, certified interpreters and oral translation programs are available. A certified interpreter, generally not a healthcare professional, may not completely understand or convey correct information. The provider needs to use terminology in nontechnical terms that the interpreter can explain to the patient.

Speak Asian

I (BA) was on duty on the postpartum unit when I received an urgent call from one of the physicians in the emergency department. He needed help with a pregnant woman. I notified my supervisor and handed off my patients to another nurse. When I arrived in the ED, the distraught physician explained that no one could talk to this woman in advanced labor, apparently of Asian origin. Knowing that I had worked extensively in "Asia," he ordered me, in a haughty, face-saving voice, "Speak Asian to this patient."

I was incredulous! "Speak Asian?" I responded. "There are hundreds of Southeast Asian languages. Let's find out where she is from."

The woman appeared to be close to giving birth. Her clothing, the traditional clothing worn by the Hmong people, was on a chair next to her. Facing the woman, I said the word "Hmong," and the woman nodded, looking very relieved. However, that did not solve the problem. I had worked in Cambodia and in the refugee camps. I knew some Thai and Khmer (Cambodia) but no Hmong. But, at that moment, she was ready to push.

She was quickly transferred to the hospital birthing center where I asked permission to stay with her. The supervisor agreed and the woman, holding firmly onto my hand, gave birth to a normal baby girl. Later, at a more auspicious time, I explained to the emergency room doctor that there are over 6,800 languages in the world and Hmong is spoken mainly in Laos and northern Thailand. He stated, "I had no idea there were that many languages in the world."

In our multicultural nation, the range of languages and even regional and cultural dialects among those speaking English or Spanish is enormous. Translation is frequently necessary but not always possible. Inability to communicate can be a significant barrier with the potential of risky misunderstandings. Overcoming linguistic barriers is one of the multicultural challenges facing the healthcare system in America.

Ageism and Extremes of Reproductive Age

At either end of childbearing age, there are increased risks. While the fertility rate has substantially decreased among adolescents over the past 20 years, it has doubled among women aged 40 to 44 and quadrupled among women greater than 45 years (Matthews & Hamilton, 2014). Overall, the very young have better outcomes than those at the upper edge of childbearing. The overall maternal mortality rate for women aged 15 to 24 is 11/100,000 compared to 38.5/100,000 for women aged 35 to 44 (CDC, 2017, 2018). Cardiovascular and coronary conditions dominate mortality at all ages (Building U.S. Capacity, 2018).

Advanced Maternal Age

A number of well-controlled research studies have identified the risks of childbearing at advanced reproductive age. McCall, Nair, and Knight (2017) attributed increased maternal mortality to five factors:

- Age greater than 35 years
- Smoking during pregnancy
- Lack of prenatal care
- Comorbidities
- Previous pregnancy complications

Severe maternal morbidity increases with advanced maternal age. A higher incidence of cesarean is one maternal outcome (Fitzpatrick, Tuffnell, Kurinczuk, & Knight, 2017; Kenny et al., 2013; Lazariu et al., 2017). After age 40, comorbidities increase, especially renal failure and acute cardiac events (Lisonkova et al., 2017). Multiple comorbidities are often present in older mothers, including hypertension, gestational diabetes, and postpartum hemorrhage. Multiple birth gestations are also more frequent in older mothers (Kenny et al., 2013).

Age as a Cultural Stressor

The age of the mother can be a cultural stressor between providers and mothers. The adolescent (age 13–17) and the very young (age 10–12) mother face a different world from the 48-year-old woman who has finally conceived using assisted reproductive technology. The societal messages are different and may reflect biases and lack of knowledge by providers. The messages of ageism can be devastating to the mother, creating an environment in which the mother may choose not to access care because of the humiliation and discrimination involved in her encounters with providers.

Both authors have had many older mothers complain about the term "advanced maternal age," stating it was discriminatory. Also, many of our pregnant adolescents have confided to us that they felt criticized by health providers for being pregnant. In examining ageism and the extremes of reproductive age, it is worth noting that the majority of the first births in the world occur to women in their adolescent years and that the trend in high-resource nations is for delayed childbearing at an older age. The pregnant woman falling in to the extremes of reproductive age is really quite normative.

Too Young or Too Old

I (BA) was on duty as a nurse in the newborn nursery the evening that the oldest mother in the history of this particular hospital gave birth. At age 55, Cecilia had conceived by assisted reproductive technology using a donor egg and her husband's sperm. She had a number of comorbidities with the pregnancy, including hypertension and gestational diabetes, but she carried the pregnancy to 39 weeks. She and her exhausted husband rested after the planned cesarean section as I cared for their beautiful baby girl. The nursery and postpartum unit were buzzing with the gossip. Comments from the staff included "She will be 75 years old when that child barely reaches adulthood" and "The child will think her parents are her grandparents." The next day Cecilia told me she had overheard some of these comments. She said she felt really hurt, as she and her husband so desired this child.

I (BA) experienced ageism when I gave birth to my first child. One of the health providers commented directly to me, "You are much too young to have a child. You should have waited until you got into your twenties."

Aghast, I asked the provider, "How old do you think I am?"

The provider responded, "You can't be a day over 16 and probably haven't even finished high school."

Was it necessary to explain? Had the provider bothered to check the chart? What purpose was served by this judgmental comment? While looking youthful, I was age 27 and had achieved a master's degree. What if I had, in fact, been the assumed age of 16? How would I have felt? Ageism and discriminatory, judgmental remarks around the appropriateness of age of childbearing continue to be a cultural stressor and a barrier to communication and care.

RACE AND RACISM

In America, the designation of "race," attributed or self-described, is a social identity, not a genetic difference per se. The designation of race does not hold up as an exclusive categorical difference in biological and genetic make-up (Babalola, Hughes, Peck, J., Murphey, 2018; Roberts, 2015; Williams, 2016). Genetic differences in individuals and populations are an expression of geographical ancestry and individual genetic configuration (Babalola et al., 2018). There are often significant differences among full-blooded siblings and even some difference between identical twins. A self-identified non-Hispanic White or African American may carry genes from a wide range of geographical ancestry. In addition, genetic expression varies according to the dominance of specific genes and the epigenetic environment that promotes gene expression. The individual genome is not one's race or ethnicity. It is part of the mosaic of an individual's life story.

Although frequently used to segment and collectively describe populations (Roberts, 2015), race or ethnicity does not maim or kill. The culprit is the pervasive influence of *racism*—overt discrimination, xenophobia, implicit bias, and assumptions about persons and groups socially identified by race or ethnicity. Living continuously in an environment that categorizes and denigrates, based upon a defined characteristic, takes its toll. This chronic stress (weathering) sets up high-alert hormonal hyperactivity (allostatic load) that undermines the health of individuals and population groups (Cheng & Solomon, 2014; Fine & Kotelchuck, 2010; Geronimus, Hicken, Keene, & Bound, 2006; Loftman, 2017; Williams, 2016).

Maternal Mortality by Race/Ethnicity

Racism is devastating to mothers of color in America. It affects health, prepregnancy comorbidities, severe maternal morbidity, and maternal mortality. Overall, African American mothers are at triple risk of pregnancy-related mortality compared to non-Hispanic White mothers, an effect that holds even among affluent, educated women of color (Amnesty International, 2011; CDC, 2017). In New York City, that risk is 12 times higher, a shocking difference in lives lost

(UNHRC, 2018). The effect of racism transcends income, education, and access to services, as highly educated women of color still have higher mortality compared to non-Hispanic Whites (Leigh & Li, 2014).

Healthcare providers may make assumptions on the basis of race. These assumptions can translate into significant differences in assigning diagnosis, providing treatment, and prescribing drugs (Williams, 2016) as well as establishing target programs. Maternal mortality by designated subpopulation or by cause of mortality provides some insight into the effects of racism but does not capture other social determinants affecting a specific group. For instance, maternal age or geography is not captured in Tables 2.2 and 2.3.

TABLE 2.2 U.S. Maternity Mortality per 100,000 Live Births by Designated Subpopulations

MATERNAL SUBPOPULATION	DEATHS PER 100,000 LIVE BIRTHS
African American	47.2
American Indian/Alaska Native	38.8
Non-Hispanic White	18.1
Hispanic	12.2
Asian-Pacific Islander	11.6

SOURCE: CDC National Vital Statistics System, 2018. Retrieved from https://www.americashealthrankings.org/explore/health-of-women-and-children/measure/maternal_mortality/state/ALL

TABLE 2.3 Leading Causes of Maternity Mortality per 100,000 Live Births: Comparing Non-Hispanic Blacks and Non-Hispanic Whites Across Nine States

CAUSE OF DEATH	NON-HISPANIC BLACKS	NON-HISPANIC WHITES
Cardiomyopathy	**1** (14%)	**5** (10.3%)
Cardiovascular/coronary	**2** (12.8%)	**1** (15.5%)
Preeclampsia/eclampsia	**3** (11.6%)	NA
Hemorrhage	**4** (10.5%)	**2** (14.4%)
Embolism	**5** (9.3%)	NA
Infection	NA	**3** (13.4%)
Mental health conditions	NA	**4** (11.3%)

SOURCE: Building U.S. Capacity to Review and Prevent Maternal Deaths. (2018). *Report from nine maternal mortality review committees.* Retrieved from http://reviewtoaction.org/Report_from_Nine_MMRCs

Severe Maternal Mortality by Race/Ethnicity

In the past 20 years, severe maternal morbidity has been rising. While the largest increase in chronic conditions has been among Asian/Pacific Islander mothers (49.1% increase; Metcalfe, Wick, & Ronksley, 2018), cardiomyopathy among African Americans is of great concern because of high mortality and disability. Closely linked to preeclampsia and eclampsia (Bello, Rendon, & Arany, 2013), cardiomyopathy disproportionally affects African American women (Howell et al., 2016; Irizarry et al., 2017; Shani et al., 2015). African American women with peripartum cardiomyopathy are sicker and more likely to die, with peak presentation of symptoms at 1 to 5 months postpartum (Irizarry et al., 2017). It is the leading cause of death and severe maternal mortality among African American mothers (Irizarry et al., 2017). The effect of racism on the epigenetics of cardiovascular health is a major factor to consider (Kuzawa & Sweet, 2009).

The Reality of My Truth

Black playwriter and producer Sharon Nyree Williams is a talented artist and a winner of the Cannes Festival Award for film production. Listen to her words on the impact of racism:

> I've worked to come to grips with who I am as a Black woman in the world, the constant battle of recognizing the beat-down in my life caused by systemic racism, questioning self-worth in the midst of recognizing the reality of my truth. (Personal communication, September 20, 2018)

Racism cripples and kills American mothers. It is one of the most damaging and deadly of the social determinants (see Box 2.1).

BOX 2.1

PHENOMENA

The backward phenomena are
That racial inequality and reproductive justice aren't intertwined,
Assumptions that the doctor knows my body better than what's in my mind,
As a woman my value is less because of my bloodline,
Life-threatening conditions aren't preventable,
Genetics and lifestyle are a death sentence,
Stress and illness have nothing to do with racial injustices in our society.

My strength allows me to fight the systemic racism that plagues me;
My beauty is beyond what man can see.
My life is worthy.
The phenomena
Just isn't me.

—Sharon Nyree Williams

MENTAL HEALTH CONDITIONS

Mental health conditions, a growing cause of pregnancy-related mortality, are also deadly. Affecting one in nine pregnant women, mental health conditions are actually treated in only 50% of those affected (CDC, 2017). Prepregnancy mental illness treated with medication can become problematic during pregnancy, as some teratogenic medications may have to be discontinued. Usually, though, the woman's medications can be adjusted during pregnancy and while lactating.

Mortality from mental health conditions is the fourth leading cause of pregnancy-related mortality among non-Hispanic White mothers (see Table 2.3). It is most likely to occur after the early postpartum period, accounting for 16.2% of all late pregnancy-related deaths from 43 to 365 days (Building U.S. Capacity, 2018). Severe maternal morbidity during the antenatal or intrapartal period may lead to depression in the postpartum (Furuta, Sandall, Cooper, & Bick, 2014). Conversely, women with depression are at higher risk for substance abuse and chronic illness prior to pregnancy, increasing maternal morbidity (Creanga et al., 2014). Adverse childhood events and posttraumatic stress may cloud the joy of having a child. Postpartum psychosis is particularly terrifying for the woman and her family, necessitating rapid protection of the baby. A sudden manifestation of bipolar disease can cause rapid psychological deterioration and violent outcomes, including suicide (Sit, Rothschild, & Wisner, 2006).

In the past 20 years, suicide rates have increased significantly in the United States, often without prior diagnosis of mental illness (Stone et al., 2018). While depression rates are lower in pregnant women than among nonpregnant women, the prevalence of depression during pregnancy is estimated at 10% to 20% (Building U.S. Capacity, 2018; Connelly, Hazen, Baker-Ericzén, Landsverk, & Horwitz, 2013; Wallace, Hoyert, Williams, & Mendola, 2016). Suicidal ideation is fairly common during pregnancy and is a risk factor for subsequent suicide in the postpartum or during the 1st year after delivery (Gelaye, Kajeepeta, & Williams, 2016). A history of depressive disorder, homelessness, lack of social support, prior suicide attempt, posttraumatic stress disorder (PTSD), bipolar disorder, and postpartum psychosis are strong risk factors for pregnancy-related suicide (Building U.S. Capacity, 2018; Gelaye et al., 2016).

An adverse social environment can contribute to the erosion of mental health during childbearing and pregnancy-related suicide (Building U.S. Capacity, 2018; Gelaye et al., 2016; Metz et al., 2016; Palladino, Singh, Campbell, Flynn, & Gold, 2011). Childhood maltreatment, childhood sexual abuse, and child rape are examples of adverse childhood experiences (ACE) that can result in PTSD and increased risk for suicide during childbearing (Bell & Seng, 2013; Leeners, Rath, Block, Görres, & Tschudin, 2014; Seng et al., 2013).

ADVERSE LIFE EXPERIENCES

Damaging or deadly for American mothers are social determinants of poverty, racism, inaccessible care, and comorbidities during pregnancy. Exposure to additional adverse life experiences is equally damaging or deadly. Some particularly detrimental experiences for maternal health are IPV, incarceration, and substance abuse.

Intimate Partner Violence

A history of ACE increases the risk of IPV during pregnancy (Huth-Bocks, Krause, Ahlfs-Dunn, Gallagher, & Scott, 2013). The occurrence of IPV is pervasive during the childbearing cycle. A large body of research describes the effects of IPV on depression, increased maternal morbidity, and serious risk for mortality from both homicide and suicide (Alhusen, Ray, Sharps, & Bullock, 2015). Mortality is double for pregnant women experiencing IPV compared to nonpregnant women (Deshpande, Kucirka, Smith, & Oxford, 2017).

IPV is implicated in over 54% of pregnancy-associated suicides and occurs most frequently among non-Hispanic White and AIAN women. With pregnancy-associated homicides, over 45% involved IPV, most often among African American women (Alhusen et al., 2015; CDC, 2018; Palladino et al., 2011; Wallace et al., 2016). The National Violent Death Reporting System (NVDRS) manages the data on violent pregnancy-associated deaths (CDC, 2018).

Incarceration

According to the Bureau of Justice Statistics, 4% of state inmates and 3% of federal inmates are pregnant at the time of incarceration. Only 54% receive any pregnancy care (Maruschak, 2019). Currently there are no national standards or evidence-based best practices in the criminal justice system that address care of pregnant and parenting women (Goshin, Arditti, Dallaire, Shlafer, & Hollihan, 2017). Pregnant women living on the streets are frequently subjected to criminalization by virtue of homelessness (UNHRC, 2018). Their choices and options for survival are limited. They often suffer from depression, PTSD, drug abuse, violence, and frequent incarceration (American Psychological Association, 2017; Crawford, Trotter, Sittner Harshorn, & Whitbeck, 2011; Sufrin, 2017). Sometimes they deliberately seek to be incarcerated just to receive food, shelter, and medical care (Sufrin, 2017). An anthropologist and obstetrician, Carolyn Sufrin exposes the realities of pregnancy in jail in her stunning work entitled *Jailcare: Finding the Safety Net for Women Behind Bars* (2017).

Once a pregnant woman is incarcerated, even if she is a nonviolent offender, she may be subjected to multiple risks to her health, her pregnancy, and the well-being of her baby. According to the Rebecca Project for Human Rights and the National Women's Law Center (NWLC; 2010), most of the states in the nation fail to provide adequate prenatal care, nutrition, HIV testing, advanced arrangements for intrapartal care, and screening for high-risk conditions.

Pregnant prisoners are frequently shackled during transport for medical care, including during labor, even if they present no flight risk or history of violent behavior. Leg irons and heavy waist restraints can present safety risks for falling. Most states have no institutional policy for justification with shackling, and guards generally have no safety training in shackling pregnant women. In most states, healthcare providers are not allowed input into decisions for shackling, even in active labor or emergent situations (Rebecca Project for Human Rights & NWLC, 2010). The Rebecca Project for Human Rights, an initiative of the NWLC, has led in the collaboration of multiple professional associations raising the issue of human rights violations with incarcerated mothers (Rebecca Project for Human Rights & NWLC, 2010). SisterSong Women of Color Reproductive Justice Collective led the campaign to stop shackling of women during childbirth in North Carolina (Turcotte, 2018).

Substance Use in Pregnancy

One of the most common factors contributing to adverse maternal outcomes is the use and abuse of both legal and illicit drugs. The U.S. Drug Enforcement Administration (DEA) categorizes drugs with potential for dependency and abuse. The schedule ranges from high potential for dependency and abuse (Schedule 1) to relatively low potential (Schedule V; DEA, n.d.). While there are many drugs that can affect maternal health, this section focuses on commonly used legal or illicit drugs of dependency and abuse.

Dependency drug use is closely associated with mental health conditions, poverty, late entry to prenatal care, poor follow-through with prenatal care, and inadequate weight gain in pregnancy (Building U.S. Capacity, 2018). With limited access to residential drug treatment for pregnant women and the criminalization of drug-addicted mothers, the safety net for treatment is very weak (UNHRC, 2018). Clinicians often struggle to provide appropriate clinic-based services.

Tobacco

Tobacco, a legal drug after adolescence, is associated with placenta previa and placental abruption, both of which can be life threatening or result in severe maternal morbidity (Creanga et al., 2014). Smoking has been attributed to increased maternal mortality among women greater than 35 years old (McCall et al., 2017). While the use of tobacco is lower among pregnant women compared to nonpregnant women (26%), it is still very high (Substance Abuse and Mental Health Services Administration [SAMHSA], 2014). In the first trimester of pregnancy, about 20% of women continue to smoke, declining to about 10% to 12% by the third trimester (CDC, 2017; SAMHSA, 2014).

Alcohol

Alcohol is also a legal drug after adolescence. The use of alcohol during pregnancy follows the pattern of tobacco use. It is higher among nonpregnant women; yet about 9.4% of pregnant women use alcohol, 2.3% binge drink, and 0.4% report heavy drinking (SAMHSA, 2014). While the direct impact is primarily on the fetus, alcohol use in pregnancy may also impact maternal health. Alcohol-related depression, accidents including falls and motor vehicle accidents, IPV, and loss of appetite for healthy foods are potential maternal risks (Villa, 2018).

Marijuana

Marijuana is in a gray zone; it is legal in some states. It is classified as a Schedule 1 drug (DEA, n.d.). The potency of marijuana today is estimated to be six to seven times stronger than it was between 1970 and 2000 (Sevigny, 2013). An estimated 11% of pregnant women use marijuana (SAMHSA, 2013). It has been shown to increase maternal anemia (Gunn et al., 2016) and promote excessive weight gain during pregnancy (Warner, Roussos-Ross, & Behnke, 2014). The full impact of marijuana on maternal health, while still not completely known, appears to be more benign than other Schedule 1 and 2 drugs.

Drugs With High Dependency Potential

The CDC Pregnancy Risk Assessment Monitoring System (PRAMS) estimates that 5% of pregnant women misuse prescribed dependency drugs or use drugs illicitly (CDC, 2017). Prescription opioid abuse is epidemic in the United States, along with a triple rise in heroin use since 2000, readily available at an affordable cost on the black market (Rudd, Aleshire, Zibbel, & Gladden, 2016).

Opioids present a particular challenge in that they are potent pain killers often prescribed in pregnancy. Supporting appropriate pain control for comorbid conditions and preventing the slide into nonmedical dependency may be a difficult judgment call for clinicians.

Heroin, methamphetamines (Schedule 1), cocaine, and opioids (Schedule 2) can be lethal to pregnant women. Placental abruption is a major concern. It can result in massive hemorrhage, shock, and disseminated intravascular coagulation. Cardiac arrest is another risk (Building U.S. Capacity, 2018; Maeda, Bateman, Clancy, Creanga, & Leffert, 2014; Metz et al., 2016). Opioid-related maternal mortality has increased 127% over the past 20 years. The prevalence continues to rise (Maeda et al., 2014).

Jamie: Without an Anchor

Jamie was unforgettable. I (BA) cared for her during her third and fourth pregnancies. She was one of my favorite midwifery patients. A tall, beautiful woman, she was close to age 25 at the time of her fourth and final pregnancy. Jamie had never met her father. He was only a name on the birth certificate. She was born in the county hospital while her incarcerated mother, a crack addict, was shackled during the birth. Her mother always reminded Jamie of how much pain that birth had caused her.

Jamie was taken from her mother shortly after birth as her mother had a prison sentence to complete. Aunt Sarah, who was single without children, offered to raise Jamie along with her older cousin, Bret, the child of another sister who lived on the streets. Aunt Sarah worked as a hotel maid. She was thrifty, provided adequately for the children, and loved them.

Jamie's mother cycled in and out of prison on a regular basis. When out of jail, she was more interested in obtaining her next hit than in visiting her daughter. When Jamie was 9 years old, Bret began to sexually abuse her on a regular basis. Aunt Sarah had just been diagnosed with advanced breast cancer and did not respond well to treatment. She died a year later.

Jamie then began to cycle through foster homes, depressed, cutting herself, experimenting with drugs on the streets, and failing miserably in school, which before she had always loved. She missed Aunt Sarah deeply and felt alone in the world. Jamie, a lost child, was on the way to becoming a lost mother. She gave birth to her first child, a boy, when she was age 15 and another, a girl, when she was 17. Both children went into the foster care system because Jamie was using methamphetamines to make it through the day. The social worker said she was neglecting the children. Jamie begged for another chance, over and over. She was in and out of drug rehab programs with conspicuous lack of success.

Then Jamie met Daren who promised her love, fidelity, and a baby. She was 10 weeks pregnant when I first saw her in the clinic. She admitted to using "just a little bit of Vicodin to help her nerves." Between the midwifery clinic and social services, she got every possible service in a porous, fragmented system. Daren came with her to her prenatal visits. She kept her appointments on the condition that I would be her midwife. I arranged my schedule accordingly.

With Daren at her side, Jamie gave birth to a beautiful 7-pound boy. She was radiant. I suggested child spacing and she agreed to use an intrauterine device (IUD) to give her body time to rest and her baby the best chance with her breast milk. For the next 2 years, she occasionally stopped by the clinic to show off her darling child. Then she made an appointment to have me take out her IUD. She was soon pregnant again and her pregnancy progressed normally.

One day she did not show up for her appointment. I called her. Her mother, out of prison now, answered, saying Daren had been killed accidently in a crossfire of gang violence. Jamie and her mother came to clinic 2 days later. Jamie was high on drugs and incoherent. The child was unclean and acting hungry. Jamie's mother announced she could not stick around any longer. She had a life to live. Social service reopened Jamie's case.

A couple of weeks later I got a message from social service, saying they needed to talk with me. We met at the clinic. They told me the child was in foster care and

Jamie was dead, a suicide by overdose. Jamie's story exemplifies how a mother was lost in a nation that lacks political will to support mental health, to care for lost children, and to ensure that all pregnant women survive and thrive.

SUMMARY

Modifying the social determinants of health that undermine maternal mortality has great potential for improving maternal health outcomes. Poverty, isolated settings, multiculturalism, and systemic racism have important implications for maternal health in America. Mental health conditions are linked to adverse life experiences, including IPV, and the social determinants of health. Increasingly, maternal health is impacted by a complex relationship between mental health, substance abuse, and incarceration.

> **WHAT IF**
>
> This section poses critical questions about the effects of social determinants on maternal health in the United States. The solutions to this national epidemic lie in interdisciplinary, imaginative conversation and problem solving. The authors invite the readers to consider these questions and add additional ones.

THE SOCIAL ENVIRONMENT: DETERMINANTS OF THE MATERNAL HEALTH CRISIS

What would be the impact on maternal health if sociocultural and economic needs of mothers were given priority consideration in the healthcare system?

How do rural isolation and geographical access factors affect maternal mortality and severe maternal morbidity outcomes in the United States?

If you could change one aspect of the social environment for childbearing in the United States, what would it be? And why?

How does political polarization affect maternal health outcomes in America?

REFERENCES

Agrawal, P. (2015). Maternal mortality and morbidity in the United States of America. *Bulletin of the World Health Organization, 93*(3), 133–208. doi:10.2471/BLT.14.148627

Agostino, M., Wilson, B., & Byfield, R. (2016). Identifying potentially preventable elements in severe adverse maternal events. *Journal of Obstetric, Gynecologic & Neonatal Nursing, 45*(6), 865–869. doi:10.1016/j.jogn.2015.12.016

Alhusen, J., Ray, E., Sharps, P., & Bullock, L. (2015). Intimate partner violence during pregnancy: Maternal and neonatal outcomes. *Journal of Women's Health, 24*(1), 100–106. doi:10.1089/jwh.2014.4872

American College of Obstetricians and Gynecologists Committee on Health Care for Underserved Women. (2014). *Health disparities in rural women* (Committee Opinion No. 586). Retrieved from https://www.acog.org/-/media/Committee-Opinions/Committee-on-Health-Care-for-Underserved-Women/co586.pdf?dmc=1&ts=20160402T0931414521

American Psychological Association. (2017). *End the use of restraints on incarcerated women and adolescents during pregnancy, labor, childbirth, and recovery.* Retrieved from https://www.apa.org/advocacy/criminal-justice/shackling-incarcerated-women.pdf

Amnesty International. (2011). *Deadly delivery: The maternal health care crisis in the USA: One-year update.* New York, NY: Author. Retrieved from https://cdn2.sph.harvard.edu/wp-content/uploads/sites/32/2017/06/deadlydeliveryoneyear.pdf

Babalola, O., Hughes, A., Peck, J., & Murphey, C. (2018, May 31). A history of race and the emerging role of genetics in primary care. *The Clinical Advisor.* Retrieved from https://www.clinicaladvisor.com/features/a-history-of-race-and-the-emerging-role-of-genetics-in-primary-care/article/769734/4

Bell, S., & Seng, J. (2013). Childhood maltreatment history, posttraumatic relational sequelae, and prenatal care utilization. *Journal of Obstetric, Gynecologic & Neonatal Nursing, 42*(4), 404–415. doi:10.1111/1552-6909.12223

Bello, N., Rendon, I., & Arany, Z. (2013). The relationship between pre-eclampsia and peripartum cardiomyopathy: A systematic review and meta-analysis. *Journal of the American College of Cardiology, 62*(18), 1715–1723. doi:10.1016/j.jacc.2013.08.717

Bice-Wigington, T., Simmons, L. A., & Huddleston-Casas, C. (2015). An ecological perspective on rural, low-income mothers' health. *Social Work in Public Health, 30*(2), 129–143. doi:10.1080/19371918.2014.969860

Braveman, P., & Gottlieb, L. (2014). The social determinants of health: It's time to consider the causes of the causes. *Public Health Reports, 129*(1 Suppl. 2), 19–31. doi:10.1177/00333549141291S206

Bridges, K. (2017). *The poverty of privacy rights.* Palo Alto, CA: Stanford University Press.

Bryant, A., Worjoloh, A., Caughey, A., & Washington, A. (2010). Racial/ethnic disparities in obstetric outcomes and care: Prevalence and determinants. *American Journal of Obstetrics and Gynecology, 202*(4), 335–343. doi:10.1016/j.ajog.2009.10.864

Building U.S. Capacity to Review and Prevent Maternal Deaths. (2018). *Report from nine maternal mortality review committees.* Retrieved from http://reviewtoaction.org/Report_from_Nine_MMRCs

Centers for Disease Control and Prevention. (n.d.). Reproductive health and the workplace. Retrieved from https://www.cdc.gov/niosh/topics/repro/pregnancyjob.html

Centers for Disease Control and Prevention. (2013). *Selecting effective interventions.* Retrieved from https://www.cdc.gov/globalhealth/healthprotection/fetp/training_modules/7/selecting-interventions_pg_final_09252013.pdf

Centers for Disease Control and Prevention. (2017). *Maternal health: Advancing the health of mothers in the 21st century.* Retrieved from https://www.cdc.gov/chronicdisease/resources/publications/aag/pdf/2016/aag-maternal-health.pdf

Centers for Disease Control and Prevention. (2018). *National vital statistics system, Maternal mortality by state.* Retrieved from https://www.americashealthrankings.org/explore/health-of-women-and-children/measure/maternal_mortality/state/ALL

Chatterji, P., & Markowitz, S. (2012). Family leave after childbirth and the mental health of new mothers. *The Journal of Mental Health Policy and Economics, 145*(2), 61–76.

Cheng, T., & Solomon, B. (2014). Translating life course theory to clinical practice to address health disparities. *Maternal and Child Health Journal, 18*(2), 389–395. doi:10.1007/s10995-013-1279-9

Connelly, C., Hazen, A., Baker-Ericzén, M., Landsverk, J., & Horwitz, S. (2013). Is screening for depression in the perinatal period enough? The co-occurrence of depression, substance abuse, and intimate partner violence in culturally diverse pregnant women. *Journal of Women's Health, 22*(10), 844–852. doi:10.1089/jwh.2012.4121

Crawford, D., Trotter, E., Sittner Harshorn, K., & Whitbeck, L. (2011). Pregnancy and mental health of young homeless women. *American Journal of Orthopsychiatry, 81*(2), 173–183. doi:10.1111/j.1939-0025.2011.01086.x

Creanga, A., Berg, C., Ko, J., Farr, S., Tong, V., Bruce, F. C., & Callaghan, W. (2014). Maternal mortality and morbidity in the United States: Where are we now? *Journal of Women's Health, 23*(1), 3–9. doi:10.1089/jwh.2013.4617

Deshpande, N., Kucirka, L., Smith, R., & Oxford, C. (2017). Pregnant trauma victims experience nearly 2-fold higher mortality compared to their nonpregnant counterparts. *American Journal of Obstetrics and Gynecology, 217*(5), 590.e1–590.e9. doi:10.1016/j.ajog.2017.08.004

Egerter, S., Braveman, P., Sadegh-Nobari, T., Grossman-Kahn, R., & Dekker, M. (2011). *Education and health. Exploring the social determinants of health* (Brief No. 5). Princeton, NJ: Robert Wood Johnson Foundation. Retrieved from https://www.rwjf.org/en/library/research/2011/05/education-matters-for-health.html

FAMILIESUSA. (2018). A 50-state look at Medicaid expansion. Retrieved from https://familiesusa.org/product/50-state-look-medicaid-expansion

Fine, A., & Kotelchuck, M. (2010) *Rethinking MCH: The life course model as an organizing framework.* Rockville, MD: Department of Health and Human Services. Retrieved from https://www.hrsa.gov/sites/default/files/ourstories/mchb75th/images/rethinkingmch.pdf

Fitzpatrick, K., Tuffnell, D., Kurinczuk, J., & Knight, M. (2017). Pregnancy at very advanced maternal age: A UK population-based cohort study. *BJOG 124*(7), 1097–1106. doi:10.1111/1471-0528.14269

Fox, L. (2017) *The supplemental poverty measure: 2016.* Retrieved from https://www.census.gov/content/dam/Census/library/publications/2017/demo/p60-261.pdf

Frieden, T. (2010). A framework for public health action: The health impact pyramid. *American Journal of Public Health, 100*(4), 590–595. doi:10.2105/AJPH.2009.185652

Furuta, M., Sandall, J., Cooper, D., & Bick, D. (2014). The relationship between severe maternal morbidity and psychological health symptoms at 6–8 weeks postpartum: A prospective cohort study in one English maternity unit. *BMC Pregnancy and Childbirth, 14*, 133. doi:10.1186/1471-2393-14-133

Gelaye, B., Kajeepeta, S., & Williams, M. (2016). Suicidal ideation in pregnancy: An epidemiological review. *Archives of Women's Mental Health, 19*(5), 741–751. doi:10.1007/s00737-016-0646-0

Geronimus, A., Hicken, M., Keene, D., & Bound, J. (2006). "Weathering" and age patterns of allostatic load scores among Blacks and Whites in the United States. *American Journal of Public Health, 96*(5), 826–833. doi:10.2105/AJPH.2004.060749

Goshin, L., Arditti, J., Dallaire, D., Shlafer, R., & Hollihan, A. (2017). An international human rights perspective on maternal criminal justice involvement in the United States. *Psychology, Public Policy, and Law, 23*(1), 53–67. doi:10.1037/law0000101

Gunn, J., Rosales, C., Center, K., Nuñez, A., Gibson, S., Christ, C., & Ehiri, J. (2016). Prenatal exposure to cannabis and maternal and child health outcomes: A systematic review and meta-analysis. *BMJ Open, 6*(4), e009986. doi:10.1136/bmjopen-2015-009986

Health Resources and Services Administration. (2015). *Child health USA 2014.* Retrieved from https://mchb.hrsa.gov/chusa13/health-services-utilization/p/barriers-to-prenatal-care.html

Howell, E., Egorova, N., Balbierz, A., Zeitlin, J., & Hebert, P. (2016). Black-White differences in severe maternal morbidity and site of care. *American Journal of Obstetrics & Gynecology, 214*(1), 122.e1–122.e7. doi:10.1016/j.ajog.2015.08.019

Hung, P., Kozhimannil, K., Casey, M., Henning-Smith, C., & Prasad, S. (2016). *State variations in the rural obstetric workforce.* Minneapolis: University of Minnesota Rural Health Research Center. Retrieved from http://rhrc.umn.edu/wp-content/uploads/2016/05/State-Variations-in-the-Rural-Obstetric-Workforce.pdf

Hung, P., Kozhimannil, K., Casey, M., & Moscovice, I. (2016). Why are obstetric units in rural hospitals closing their doors? *Health Services Research, 51*(4), 1546–1560. doi:10.1111/1475-6773.12441

Huth-Bocks, A., Krause, K., Ahlfs-Dunn, S., Gallagher, E., & Scott, S. (2013). Relational trauma and posttraumatic stress symptoms among pregnant women. *Psychodynamic Psychiatry, 41*(2), 277–301. doi:10.1521/pdps.2013.41.2.277

Irizarry, O., Levine, L., Lewey, J., Boyer, T., Riis, V., Elovitz, M., & Arany, Z. (2017). Comparison of clinical characteristics and outcomes of peripartum cardiomyopathy between African American and non–African American women. *JAMA Cardiology, 2*(11), 1256–1260. doi:10.1001/jamacardio.2017.3574

Kenny, L., Lavender, T., McNamee, R., O'Neill, S., Mills, T., & Khashan, A. (2013). Advanced maternal age and adverse pregnancy outcome: Evidence from a large contemporary cohort. *PLoS ONE, 8*(2), e56583. doi:10.1371/journal.pone.0056583

Kozhimannil, K., Henning-Smith, C., Hung, P., Casey, M., & Prasad, S. (2016). Ensuring access to high-quality maternity care in rural America. *Women's Health Issues, 26*, 247–250. doi:10.1016/j.whi.2016.02.001

Kuzawa, C., & Sweet, E. (2009). Epigenetics and the embodiment of race: Developmental origins of US racial disparities in cardiovascular health. *American Journal of Human Biology, 21*(1), 2–15. doi:10.1002/ajhb.20822

Lazariu, V., Nguyen, T., McNutt, L.-A., Jeffrey, J., & Kacica, M. (2017). Severe maternal morbidity: A population-based study of an expanded measure and associated factors. *PLoS ONE, 12*(8), e0182343. doi:10.1371/journal.pone.0182343

Leeners, B., Rath, W., Block, E., Görres, G., & Tschudin, S. (2014). Risk factors for unfavorable pregnancy outcome in women with adverse childhood experiences. *Journal of Perinatal Medicine, 42*(2), 171–178. doi:10.1515/jpm-2013-0003

Leigh, W. A., & Li, Y. (2014). *Women of color health data book* (4th ed.). Bethesda, MD: National Institutes of Health.

Lisonkova, S., Potts, J., Muraca, G., Razaz, N., Sabr, Y., Chan, W.-S., & Kramer, M. (2017). Maternal age and severe maternal morbidity: A population-based retrospective cohort study. *PLoS Medicine, 14*(5), e1002307. doi:10.1371/journal.pmed.1002307

Loftman, P. (2017). Racial and ethnic disparities in birth outcomes: The challenge to midwives. In B. Anderson, J. Rooks, & R. Barroso (Eds.), *Best practices in midwifery: Using the evidence to implement change* (2nd ed., pp. 183–198). New York, NY: Springer Publishing Company.

Maeda, A., Bateman, B., Clancy, C., Creanga, A., & Leffert, L. (2014). Opioid abuse and dependence during pregnancy: Temporal trends and obstetrical outcomes. *Anesthesiology, 121*(6), 1158–1165.

Markus, A., Andres, E., West, K., Garro, N., & Pellegrini, C. (2013). Medicaid covered births, 2008 through 2010, in the context of the implementation of health reform. *Women's Health Issues, 23*(5), e273–e280. doi:10.1016/j.whi.2013.06.006

Maruschak, L. (2019). Medical problems of prisoners. *Bureau of Justice Statistics.* Retrieved from https://www.bjs.gov/content/pub/html/mpp/mpp.cfm

Maternal Mortality and Morbidity Task Force & Department of State Health Services. (2016). *Joint biennial report.* Retrieved from https://dshs.texas.gov/Consumerand ExternalAffairs/legislative/2016Reports/M3TFBiennialReport2016-7-15.pdf

Matthews, T., & Hamilton, B. (2014). *First births to older women continue to rise* (NCHS Data Brief No. 152). Hyattsville, MD: National Center for Health Statistics. Retrieved from https://www.cdc.gov/nchs/data/databriefs/db152.pdf

McCall, S., Nair, M., & Knight, M. (2017). Factors associated with maternal mortality at advanced maternal age: A population-based case-control study. *BJOG: An International Journal of Obstetrics & Gynaecology, 124*(8), 1225–1232. doi:10.1111/1471 -0528.14216

Metcalfe, A., Wick, J., & Ronksley, P. (2018). Racial disparities in comorbidity and severe maternal morbidity/mortality in the United States: An analysis of temporal trends. *Acta Obstetricia et Gynecologica Scandinavica, 97*(1), 89–96. doi:10.1111/aogs.13245

Metz, T., Royner, P., Hoffman, M., Allshouse, A., Beckwith, K., & Binswanger, I. (2016). Maternal deaths from suicide and overdose in Colorado, 2004–2012. *Obstetrics and Gynecology, 128*(6), 1233–1240. doi:10.1097/AOG.0000000000001695

Natamba, B., Mehta, S., Achan, J., Stoltzfus, R., Griffiths, J., & Young, S. (2017). The association between food insecurity and depressive symptoms severity among pregnant women differs by social support category: A cross-sectional study. *Maternal & Child Nutrition, 13*(3), e12351. doi:10.1111/mcn.12351

Neckermann, C. (2017). An international embarrassment: The United States as an anomaly in maternity leave policy. *Harvard International Review, 38*(4), 36–39. Retrieved from http://hir.harvard.edu/archive/?s=Christina%20Neckermann

Palladino, C., Singh, V., Campbell, J., Flynn, H., & Gold, K. (2011). Homicide and suicide during the perinatal period: Findings from the National Violent Death Reporting System. *Obstetrics and Gynecology, 118*(5), 1056–0163. doi:10.1097/AOG.0b013e31823294da

Plotka, R., & Busch-Rossnagel, N. (2018). The role of length of maternity leave in supporting mother–child interactions and attachment security among American mothers and their infants. *International Journal of Child Care and Education Policy, 12*(1), 2. doi:10.1186/s40723-018-0041-6

Rebecca Project for Human Rights & National Women's Law Center. (2010). *Mothers behind bars.* Washington, DC: National Women's Law Center. Retrieved from http://www.rebeccaprojectjustice.org/images/stories/files/mothersbehindbarsreport-2010.pdf

Redden, M. (2016). Texas has highest maternal mortality rate in developed world, study finds. *The Guardian.* Retrieved from https://www.theguardian.com/us-news/2016/aug/20/texas-maternal-mortality-rate-health-clinics-funding

Roberts, D. (2015). *The problem with race-based medicine* [Video file]. Retrieved from https://www.ted.com/talks/dorothy_roberts_the_problem_with_race_based_medicine?utm_source=tedcomshare&utm_medium=email&utm_campaign=tedspread

Rudd, R. A., Aleshire, N., Zibbel, J. E., & Gladden, R. M. (2016). Increases in drug and opioid overdose deaths—United States, 2000–2014. *Morbidity and Mortality Weekly Report, 64*(50), 1378–1382. Retrieved from https://www.cdc.gov/mmwr/preview/mmwrhtml /mm6450a3.htm

Seng, J., Sperlich, M., Low, L., Ronis, D., Muzik, M., & Liberzon, I. (2013). Childhood abuse history, posttraumatic stress disorder, postpartum mental health, and bonding: A prospective cohort study. *Journal of Midwifery & Women's Health, 58*(1), 57–68. doi:10.1111/j.1542-2011.2012.00237.x

Sevigny, E. (2013). Is today's marijuana more potent simply because it's fresher? *Drug Testing and Analysis, 5*(1), 62–67. doi:10.1002/dta.1430

Shani, H., Kuperstein, R., Berlin, A., Arad, M., Goldenberg, I., & Simchen, M. (2015). Peripartum cardiomyopathy—Risk factors, characteristics and long-term follow-up. *Journal of Perinatal Medicine, 43*(1), 95–101. doi:10.1515/jpm-2014-0086

Sit, D., Rothschild, A., & Wisner, K. (2006). A review of postpartum psychosis. *Journal of Women's Health, 15*(4), 352–368. doi:10.1089/jwh.2006.15.352

Stone, D., Simon, T., Fowler, K., Kegler, S., Yuan, K., Holland, K., . . . Crosby, A. (2018, June 8). Vital signs: Trends in state suicide rates—United States, 1999–2016 and circumstances contributing to suicide—27 States, 2015. *Morbidity and Mortality Weekly Report, 67*(22), 617–624. doi:10.15585/mmwr.mm6722a1

Substance Abuse and Mental Health Services Administration. (2013). *Results from the 2012 National Survey on Drug Use and Health: Summary of national findings* (NSDUH Series H-46, HHS Publication No. (SMA) 13-4795). Rockville, MD: Author. Retrieved from https://www.samhsa.gov/data/sites/default/files/NSDUHresults2012/NSDUHresults2012.pdf

Substance Abuse and Mental Health Services Administration. (2014). *Results from the 2013 National Survey on Drug Use and Health: Summary of national findings* (NSDUH Series H-48, HHS Publication No. (SMA) 14-4863). Rockville, MD: Author. Retrieved from   https://www.samhsa.gov/data/sites/default/files/NSDUHresultsPDFWHTML2013/Web/NSDUHresults2013.pdf

Sufrin, C. (2017). *Jailcare: Finding the safety net for women behind bars*. Oakland: University of California Press.

Tilden, V., Cox, K., Moore, J., & Naylor, M. (2018). Strategic partnerships to address adverse social determinants of health: Redefining health care. *Nursing Outlook, 66*(3), 233–236. doi:10.1016/j.outlook.2018.03.002

Turcotte, M. (2018, April 24). What's next in the fight for reproductive justice for incarcerated women? *Ms. Magazine*. Retrieved from http://msmagazine.com/blog/2018/04/24/the-fight-to-protect-pregnant-women-from-being-shackled-in-north-carolina-prisons-and-across-the-u-s

Ungar, L. (2018, September 20). What states aren't doing to save new mothers' lives. *USA Today*. Retrieved from https://www.usatoday.com/in-depth/news/investigations/deadly-deliveries/2018/09/19/maternal-death-rate-state-medical-deadly-deliveries/547050002

United Nations Human Rights Council. (2018). *Report of the Special Rapporteur on extreme poverty and human rights on his mission to the United States of America*. Retrieved from https://digitallibrary.un.org/record/1629536/files/A_HRC_38_33_Add-1-EN.pdf

United Nations Population Fund. (2012). *Rich mother, poor mother: The social determinants of maternal death and disability*. Retrieved from https://www.unfpa.org/sites/default/files/resource-pdf/EN-SRH%20fact%20sheet-Poormother.pdf

United States Drug Enforcement Administration. (n.d.). Drug scheduling. Retrieved from https://www.dea.gov/drug-scheduling

U.S. Department of Agriculture Economic Research Service. (2018). *Rural American at a glance: 2018 edition*. Retrieved from https://www.ers.usda.gov/webdocs/publications/90556/eib-200.pdf?v=5899.2

U.S. Department of Agriculture Economic Research Service. (2019). Population and migration: Overview. Retrieved from http://www.ers.usda.gov/topics/rural-economy-population/population-migration.aspx

U.S. Department of Health and Human Services, Health Resources and Services Administration Maternal and Child Health Bureau. (2011). Women's health USA 2011. Retrieved from http://mchb.hrsa.gov/whusa11

Vance, J. (2016). *Hillbilly elegy: A memoir of a family and culture in crisis*. New York, NY: HarperCollins.

Villa, L. (2018). Dangers of drinking while pregnant. *DrugAbuse.com*. Retrieved from https://drugabuse.com/library/drinking-while-pregnant

Wallace, M., Hoyert, D., Williams, C., & Mendola, P. (2016). Pregnancy-associated homicide and suicide in 37 US states with enhanced pregnancy surveillance. *American Journal of Obstetrics and Gynecology, 215*(3), 364.e1–364.e10. doi:10.1016/j.ajog.2016.03.040

Warner, T., Roussos-Ross, D., & Behnke, M. (2014). It's not your mother's marijuana: Effects on maternal-fetal health and the developing child. *Clinics in Perinatology, 41*(4), 877–894. doi:10.1016/j.clp.2014.08.009

Williams, D. (2016) How racism makes us sick [Video file]. Retrieved from https://www.ted .com/talks/david_r_williams_how_racism_makes_us_sick?utm_source=tedcom share&utm_medium=email&utm_campaign=tedspread

World Health Organization. (n.d.). *Social determinants of health*. Retrieved from http:// www.who.int/social_determinants/en

THE LIVED EXPERIENCE OF CHILDBEARING

The Lifelong Impact

LISA R. ROBERTS

At the end of this chapter, the reader will be able to:

1. Examine the influence of prior life experiences, as they affect childbearing outcome.

2. Describe how childbearing experiences and outcomes can have a lifelong impact.

3. Discuss how health professionals can use life course theory to evaluate undermining social determinants affecting childbearing outcome.

THE LIFELONG IMPACT OF CHILDBEARING

All of a woman's prior life experiences and her individual way of facing these experiences influence how she approaches childbearing. Whether pregnancy is planned or unintended, relished or endured, birth is a turning point. An empowering birth, supportive, respectful care even with complications or a near miss, abusive treatment during birth, severe maternal morbidity, or perinatal loss will never be forgotten. Her journey of childbearing, no matter the outcome or how many times it occurs, becomes a part of the fabric of her being for the remainder of her life (King & Pinger, 2014).

The Mantle of Motherhood

Allison, a nursing professor and public health educator, was teaching maternal–child health in a graduate public health program. She was also a single mother, raising two children. In her classes, she frequently discussed the joys of parenting, the stresses of work–life balance, and the influence of motherhood on her life course. Students who had children or became parents after graduation frequently brought their children to her office for her admiration. One day a former student brought her newborn child to Allison's office. There was much cooing and delight by the mother, the professor, and the department secretary. As Allison cradled the infant in her arms, the secretary remarked, "Allison would have been such a good mother."

The former student and the professor looked up at the secretary in surprise. "But I am a mother," said Allison.

Nonplused, the secretary continued, "But you aren't really a family since you have a broken home." This was a profoundly negative message about the social and historical environment of motherhood in America.

Allison, knowing this was a teachable moment, at least for the former student, quietly explained that there are many ways to make a family and that motherhood comes in many forms. Later Allison had two experiences that cemented this belief. First, she remarried and, with her new partner, formed a blended family, parenting more children. Secondly, in her faculty practice as a patient educator, she cared for a severely alcoholic pregnant woman who drank up to 24 beers each day. Melissa was 14 weeks pregnant when she requested an abortion. She wanted help with the alcoholism, knew she had hurt her child, and did not want her child to suffer. Then, in great anguish, she said, "But I always wanted to be a mother." Another teachable moment about the mantle of motherhood.

"But you are a mother, Melissa," Allison told her. "That will never change; you are forever a mother. You will always know that you held this child in your womb and that you cared for your little one, making what you believe is your best decision. Your child will always be with you."

Melissa chose to have an abortion and then entered rehabilitation. She told the alcohol rehabilitation counselor that she was a mother now and had to get healthy so maybe in the future she could have a healthy child. She wore the mantle of motherhood as part of her lived experience and it became her strength.

Childbearing and Life Course Theory

A mother's health, at any given point, is shaped by prior health and life experiences (United Nations Population Fund, 2012; World Health Organization [WHO], n.d.-a, n.d.-b), underscoring the critical impact of the social determinants of health, that is, poverty, geographical isolation, racism, mental illness, and adverse life experiences. High maternal mortality and severe morbidity in the United States are linked to the poorer health and shorter lives of Americans compared to counterparts in other developed nations (Building U.S. Capacity to Review and Prevent Maternal Deaths, 2018; United Nations Human Rights Council [UNHRC], 2018; Woolf & Aron, 2013).

One means of examining childbearing outcomes is through using life course theory, a holistic framework that enables clinical and public health professionals to identify undermining social determinants and life events. It is a useful tool in evaluating the impact of health disparity and inequity (Cheng & Solomon, 2014; Halfon & Hochstein, 2002) and it is applicable to critical thinking about determinants of maternal health, mortality, and morbidity (Fine & Kotelchuck, 2010; Miesnik & Stringer, 2002). It can provide excellent data for the Pregnancy Risk Assessment Monitoring System (PRAMS), the Centers for Disease Control and Prevention (CDC) surveillance project that evaluates maternal attitudes before, during, and after pregnancy (CDC, n.d.; Wyoming Department of Health, n.d).

Key overarching themes in life course theory are the importance of the physical body and the inseparability of mind and body (Black, Holditch-Davis, & Miles, 2009). Life course theory maps two key concepts, the *trajectory of a person's life* and *transitions to new life experiences*, utilizing five principles: context, developmental stage, timing, agency, and linked lives (Black et al., 2009). These principles are further described in the following sections.

Context

Sociohistorical and geographical location are the major components of context, which consider geopolitical events (e.g., mass immigration), economic cycles (e.g., the great recession of the last decade), and sociocultural norms (e.g., patriarchal societal structure). Context shapes families' and individuals' behaviors and decision making (Alwin, 2012). Understanding context informs understanding of mothers. For instance, exposure to domestic violence as a young child, such as witnessing her mother's abuse, may not have any obvious effect until a woman becomes a mother herself. The early exposure shapes her attitude toward women, violence, and motherhood (Mortimer & Shanahan, 2003).

Developmental Stage

Developmental stages include infancy, early childhood, school age, adolescence, young adulthood, middle adulthood, and older adulthood. Both psychosocial processes and physical growth are milestones that typically mark these developmental stages. Early life events, cultural and environmental exposures, and both mental and physical health have major implications for risk and protection across all developmental stages of a woman's life. Significant psychosocial and/or physiologic stress experienced at any developmental stage can affect maternal health and birth outcomes (Allen, Feinberg, & Mitchell, 2014; Halfon, Larson, Lu, Tullis, & Russ, 2014).

Timing

Individual age encompasses both chronological age and age-related changes (aging). Perceived deadlines for transitions such as educational attainment, moving out of the family home, marriage, and parenting are important aspects of timing. Timing and perceived deadlines are individually variable and may or may not be flexible. Another aspect of timing is generational. Generations are age groups or cohorts based on age in a given time, such as Baby Boomers (1946–1964), Generation X (1965–1980), Millennials (1981–1997), and Post-Millennials (born after 1997). Timing also encompasses each generation's reaction to the sociohistorical time in which they live, creating a cohort effect. Sociohistorical time (historical time related to social changes) is defined by large-scale changes, such as the information age (Internet), which affects the population across individual age and generation. Subjective experience of large-scale social structures and changes influence one's life course (Alwin, 2012; Mortimer & Shanahan, 2003).

Agency

Individuals are active decision makers within opportunities and constraints, available or perceived. "Agency" is the concept of personal control. Planning, modification of expectations, and adaptive behavior in response to circumstances shape the construction of one's biography. Self-efficacy, intellect, effort, a sense of personal responsibility, and context are components of agency. Individuals with high levels of self-efficacy are likely to view their lives with an internal locus of control (perspective of having influence over their own destiny), whereas those with low self-efficacy are likely to view their lives with an external locus of control (victims of circumstance, fatalistic view). Perceived agency, or the lack of it, can be either protective or risk producing across women's life course (Alwin, 2012; Mortimer & Shanahan, 2003).

Linked Lives

Social ties form a network of shared relationships. Due to the nature of interdependent, reciprocal relationships, major changes affecting one member of the network (death, divorce, job loss, etc.) have a ripple effect throughout the network. Supporting one another reinforces ties and promotes collective well-being. Tension between individual goals and collective needs may have a destructive effect on the network (Alwin, 2012). Social integration connects individual lives across generations, linking older and younger family members. Women are likely to construct their biographies based on linked lives. Women frequently consider the needs of husband/children/parents in their decision making related to time allocations and roles at work and in their private lives (Mortimer & Shanahan, 2003).

Life course theory further examines a third concept, *turning points*, identifying the effect of life events from the perspective of the five principles (Black et al., 2009).

Applicability to Childbearing Women

This theory has applicability for health professionals working with childbearing women (Miesnik & Stringer, 2002; Black et al., 2009). Adverse childbearing

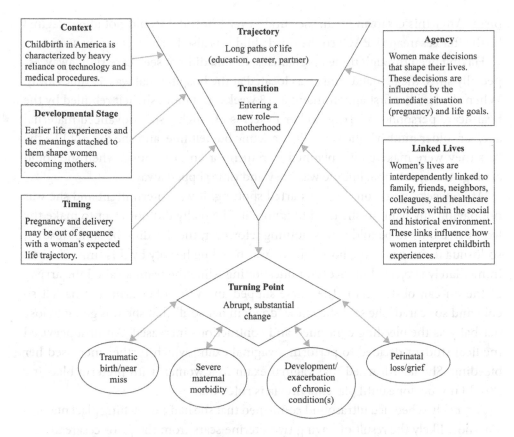

Context

Childbirth in America is characterized by heavy reliance on technology and medical procedures.

Developmental Stage

Earlier life experiences and the meanings attached to them shape women becoming mothers.

Timing

Pregnancy and delivery may be out of sequence with a woman's expected life trajectory.

Trajectory

Long paths of life (education, career, partner)

Transition

Entering a new role— motherhood

Agency

Women make decisions that shape their lives. These decisions are influenced by the immediate situation (pregnancy) and life goals.

Linked Lives

Women's lives are interdependently linked to family, friends, neighbors, colleagues, and healthcare providers within the social and historical environment. These links influence how women interpret childbirth experiences.

Turning Point

Abrupt, substantial change

Traumatic birth/near miss

Severe maternal morbidity

Development/ exacerbation of chronic condition(s)

Perinatal loss/grief

FIGURE 3.1 Life course theory applied to adverse childbearing outcomes.

outcomes provide examples of turning points in a woman's life trajectory. Figure 3.1 applies the theoretical framework of the life course theory to selected situations resulting in adverse childbearing outcomes. The following exemplars use life course theory to describe the trajectory, the transition, and the turning points for women experiencing adverse childbearing outcomes.

FOUR MOTHERS: TRAJECTORY, TRANSITION, TURNING POINT

No Time to Lose

Joshua and Emma had a family farm in the rural Midwest. They had three healthy daughters, the last two born by cesarean section. At age 43, Emma was surprised to learn she was pregnant again. Though unplanned, she and her husband took the pregnancy in stride and soon warmed to the idea of another little one. Their daughters were delighted and together the family prepared for the arrival of the baby. Emma was a physically active woman who had experienced three full-term pregnancies. The first birth was vaginal but the second was breech with cesarean birth. After this cesarean birth, the rural Level 1 hospital would not allow vaginal birth after cesarean (VBAC) so the third child was also born by cesarean section.

Having been through three pregnancies, Emma did not seek care right away, especially since the prenatal clinic was located at the hospital that was 50 miles away. When she had her first appointment at 18 weeks' gestation, she felt rebuffed by the healthcare personnel referring to her in terms of "high risk," "advanced maternal age," or "older mother." She was a little anemic but felt fine, and she did not like the fuss they were making. She planned to return for an ultrasound when she could arrange transportation, but life was busy and time slipped away.

At 26 weeks' gestation, Emma started spotting. It was intermittent and she was not having any pain, so she tried to ignore it. She really did not want to make the long drive only to be told it was nothing. However, the bleeding became steadier, so Joshua drove her to the hospital. She was bleeding heavily by this time. She was immediately subjected to incessant questioning while the team awaited the arrival of the on-call obstetrician. The nurse slipped an IV into her arm. Emma felt so cold and so scared. She said she knew "down in her soul" that she was going to lose her baby as the bleeding continued and contractions increased. An unsupervised medical student decided to perform a vaginal exam, which further increased her bleeding. She later learned that vaginal exam in a woman with preterm bleeding should not be done until placenta previa is ruled out.

A quickly scheduled ultrasound confirmed that she had a detaching placenta previa, most likely the result of having two uterine scars from the prior cesarean sections. The on-call obstetrician arrived and an emergency cesarean section quickly followed. Her tiny baby boy needed immediate transport to a higher level of neonatal intensive care as this hospital had only basic support services for compromised neonates. The infant succumbed before arrangements could be completed.

Emma wanted little else but to have her family gathered around her and to hold her dying baby. Instead, there seemed to be blood everywhere, in pools under her and in transfusion lines above her. Blood transfusions followed one after another, amid calls for more blood. The medical jargon seemed to depersonify her and her baby. Being talked about as though she were not in the room interrupted her dimming thoughts while she tried to grapple with the situation. Her head began to spin and she felt very cold. Everything happened so fast.

The next thing Emma remembers is waking up in the intensive care unit. She was on oxygen, had a urinary catheter, an IV, and a unit of blood running. Opening her eyes, she gazed at Joshua, sitting beside her, looking anxious and relieved at the same time. His tears flowed as he explained that it had been a near miss, a massive hemorrhage. He explained that she had gone unconscious, her organs were shutting down, and he had consented to the lifesaving hysterectomy. Emma remembers the kind eyes of the nurse who explained disseminating intravascular coagulation (DIC) to her. Later the nurse brought the baby to the couple, his tiny face now set in the death mask. Joshua and Emma named him Brandon and held him close to their hearts. Emma became very fatigued and emotional. The nurse suggested that she take the baby back to morgue for the time being. Looking back on her experience, Emma said she wished she had spoken up to limit the overwhelming questioning when she first arrived at the hospital and she also wished she had been able to hold her little son longer.

Although Emma's pregnancy was unexpected, it was not incongruent with her life trajectory. She was transitioning seamlessly to being a mother of four. The untoward timing of her labor and the emergent nature of the situation diminished Emma's sense of agency. She said, "Things were just happening. There were no decisions." Joshua said he felt overwhelmed by having to make a huge decision with Emma unconscious and unable to participate, but he is so grateful that his wife is alive. Emma described her lived experience as traumatic, "There was so much blood. It was everywhere, soaked through everything. I can still see it, smell it. . . ." Now 6 years later, Emma still cries when she talks about the little boy she lost. She gets upset, even angry, when she talks about her hospital experience. "If it hadn't been for that wonderful nurse who explained everything and brought Brandon for me to hold…," she continues. She admits that thoughts of her near miss haunt her but that she feels fortunate to be alive, to be with Joshua and her growing family.

Ghosts of the Past

Jenny grew up in a trailer park. Her father was an alcoholic, out of work most of the time. Her mother worked two jobs, trying to keep the family afloat. When she was a child, Jenny was lonely and had longed for siblings. As an adolescent, she was called "white trash" (see Isenberg, 2017). She was determined to leave as soon as she could and to make something of herself. She went to community college but did not finish the program because she met the love of her life. They soon married and she got a job at a local diner. She laughs saying, "My life sounds like a country love song." She quickly sobers, however, saying everything changed when she got pregnant. She battled anxiety and depression throughout the pregnancy. She feared that she would lose her job and that she would end up back in a trailer park. Her manager was already harassing her about missing work for prenatal appointments. It did not help that one day she had to leave work due to a panic attack.

Low-income women often face severe poverty if they have a child. A pervasive lack of social support discourages women from childbearing. In 2015, according to the Department of Labor, 25% of new mothers returned to work within 2 weeks of giving birth. The lack of paid leave is a major contributor to early return to work, as a woman may have no financial choice, despite detrimental health consequences for her and her newborn (Peck, 2018).

Higher income mothers are often passed over for promotions and raises and are subjected to greater scrutiny than others in terms of punctuality and attendance. They also face other biases, such as an assumption that they are not dedicated to their work (Peck, 2018). It is no wonder that career women are more likely to delay childbearing, even if it means relying on high-priced, high-technology family planning and assisted reproductive technology at the margins of childbearing potential (Simoni, Mu, & Collins, 2017). Women are caught up in the tension between choosing motherhood despite career consequences and running out of time biologically (Birch Petersen et al., 2016; Simoni et al., 2017).

Stress and depression pose significant health risk for childbearing women (Owens & Jackson, 2015). Chronic stress increases allopathic load, causing physiologic deterioration. In pregnant women, experiencing psychologic stress is associated with higher norepinephrine and cortisol levels, which causes release of placental corticotropin-releasing hormone in response to physiologic stress (Geronimus, Hicken, Keene, & Bound, 2006; Loftman, 2017; Wadhwa et al., 2004). This becomes a vicious cycle affecting both mental and physical maternal health.

As Jenny's pregnancy progressed, she resented having to ask her husband for household help. She began to see him as a loafer like her father. She dismally predicted that she would be no more connected to her child than her work-weary mother and would ultimately "fail motherhood." Negative maternal attitudes are a significant risk factor for perinatal and postpartum depression (Sockol & Battle, 2015).

Jenny could not get these thoughts out of her head. They only worsened after her daughter was born. The baby blues turned into serious postpartum depression. At the age of 23, she felt like an utter failure. After being home with her baby for 1 month and with mounting financial pressures, she decided to return to work. Instead she attempted suicide. She was barely conscious when the neighbor, who was babysitting her daughter, found her. Jenny had forgotten to pack the pacifier in the diaper bag and the neighbor came back to see if Jenny was still home so that she could get it. She found Jenny sitting in the garage, with the car exhaust running. Fortunately, the paramedics came before it was too late.

Suicidality (completion/attempts/ideation/thoughts of self-harm) is currently one of the leading causes of maternal mortality within the 1st year postpartum (Orsolini et al., 2016). Jenny had a number of risk factors but had not been adequately assessed for suicidality. A thorough assessment for perinatal suicidality risk would have included a specific screening for suicidality, such as the Scale for Suicide Ideation (SSI), the Columbia-Suicide Severity Rating Scale (C-SSRS), or the Suicide Probability Scale (SPS), in addition to general mental health screening, which most likely would have revealed her severe postpartum depression (Orsolini et al., 2016).

Although she got help, her marriage was never the same. Her daughter is a teenager now, and the typical adolescent tensions are too much for her to manage. Jenny retreats from the stress, confiding, "I'm just a shell of what I was going to be, what I set out to be, that is. Or maybe I was only fooling myself and am fulfilling my original destiny."

Jenny was ready to succeed in her life goals. However, her transition to the role of motherhood was fraught with mental health issues, perhaps due to the meanings attached to motherhood shaped by earlier life experiences. Mental health issues affected her ability to make decisions about day-to-day life, ultimately impacting her marriage and the parenting of her teenage daughter. Though her husband has stood by her, their relationship is strained. She noted, "I was a go-getter when we met. He probably wonders whatever happened to that girl." Nonetheless, she expressed gratitude for his support, stating, "He's my rock." She admitted to being plagued by a sense of failure and emptiness and continues to struggle with depression.

A New Beginning

Intimate partner violence (IPV) affects women at every socioeconomic level (Bermele, Andresen, & Urbanski, 2018; Kothari et al., 2016). Women who are victims of IPV may have diminished self-determination and reproductive decision-making power because their abusing partner often exercises extreme power and control, especially over their reproductive life (Bianchi, 2016).

Sarah, a successful real estate agent, had been married to Tom, a local businessman, for 2 years. To all outside appearances, their life together looked perfect. Except that it was not. They had a whirlwind courtship and short engagement with Tom planning their dates carefully. Sarah felt a bit stifled by his control over their activities, but she was flattered by his attention. Tom had a bad temper, which showed up once during their engagement. He abjectly apologized, bringing her flowers and promising it would not happen again.

As soon as they were married, Tom was increasingly threatened by Sarah's professional success or anything that occupied her except for catering to him. He attempted to block phone calls with her family and even his mother, whom Sarah loved very much. Tom had been an occasional drinker before the marriage, but since their marriage, his drinking became heavy. Sarah often found alcohol hidden in the closets. When she attempted to discuss this with him, he flew into a rage.

Nonetheless, she had made a commitment and she loved him. Besides, she was 32 years old and felt it was time to begin a family. Before they married, they had agreed to have two children after they got established. Now Tom announced he did not want any children. Any discussion of the issue escalated into verbal abuse by Tom and Sarah felt betrayed. Then one day, he shoved her. She dismissed it, saying, "It wasn't much. I didn't get hurt. He was really sorry and I was sure it wouldn't happen again." But it did.

Sarah was on birth control pills. When she and Tom took a short vacation, she forgot to take the pills. He was very angry when she told him, but they stopped at a pharmacy to get condoms. Later that month, Sarah missed her period and began to feel nauseous. She wondered if she was pregnant. A home pregnancy test confirmed that she was. Feeling really happy, she was sure Tom would get used to the idea. When she told him, he looked at her coldly and said, "Get an abortion." Sarah refused.

Verbal and physical abuse escalated during the pregnancy. She had occasional bruises, he used icy coldness as a weapon, and he continued drinking heavily, angry that she would not join him. Sarah felt very sad but convinced herself it would be different after the baby was born. She tried to talk to her doctor who always seemed too busy and tired to discuss anything. When Sarah went into labor, Tom took her to the hospital and dropped her off at the emergency room exit. She told him she would see him after he got parked. That was the last she saw him for the next week.

Now in active labor, she met Melissa, her labor and delivery nurse. Melissa was her lifeline during the 11-hour labor. After the birth, Melissa promised to stop by the next day. When she entered the room, Sarah was crying, trying to breastfeed the baby. Melissa helped her with the baby's latch and then sat down, quietly saying, "I knew something was really bothering you during labor, Sarah. Do you want to tell me about it?"

This was the first time Sarah felt she could open up about the escalating violence at home. Melissa gave her the permission she needed to tell Tom's mother about the situation. Tom's mother was already on the road, on her way to help with her new grandchild. When Sarah explained the situation, her mother-in-law did not seem surprised. She stayed with the couple for the next 4 months as Sarah recovered from childbirth and prepared to go back to work. Tom held the baby once and sulked when Sarah seemed tired or busy caring for the baby. His mother tried to talk to him, but he refused. She acted as the buffer when Tom's temper flared and she supported Sarah's decision to leave the marriage. The transition to motherhood escalated the IPV and caused the marriage to further deteriorate.

A Broken Heart

When Darren was offered an excellent job, Tony and Darren moved from the South, where they had deep family roots, to a midsized town in a western state. Although there were few African American families in the community and relations were cordial, racism was often implicit. Tony gave birth to her first child in this community, away from her mother, sister, and large extended family. She often wonders if racism and lack of family support were the real reasons things went so badly when she gave birth. Allopathic stress from lifelong and current racism, even if implicit, and lack of social support are key factors in adverse outcomes in childbearing (see Hutchison and Thomas, 2017; Loftman, 2017).

She had attended her prenatal visits regularly, read all the pamphlets given to her, and followed instructions from her doctor. While no childbirth education classes were offered, Tony felt she received attentive care and enjoyed socializing with other mothers in the waiting room. At 27 weeks pregnant, her blood pressure shot up. She was sent home with instructions to rest and return in 1 week. Then she started to have contractions. She called her doctor immediately. He told her to go to the hospital where he would meet her.

Tony arrived at the hospital but was told her doctor had another patient and the family practice doctor on duty would see her as soon as possible. She was apprehensive, but staff reassured her that everything would be fine. She began to wonder if it was false labor. She waited for 3 hours. Finally, she thought, "What am I doing here?" and decided to go home. "They told me if I left it would be AMA—I didn't really know what that meant, but they were not doing anything for me anyway, so I left."

At home, the pain progressively worsened and the contractions were more frequent. Tony wondered if this was the "real thing" after all, but her water did not break and she did not have the "show" she had read about in the pamphlets. She did have a bad headache and her ankles seemed very swollen. She tried to be calm. If this was false labor, she could not imagine how painful actual labor would be. In desperation, she called her mother, who told her to call an ambulance. Instead she called Darren who took her back to the hospital.

When they arrived at the hospital, Tony's blood pressure was 170/95 and fetal monitoring indicated the baby was in distress. With limited explanation to Darren and Tony, the doctor said they must do an emergency cesarean section. As soon as their tiny baby was born, he was whisked off to the neonatal intensive care unit. Tony recalls, "The doctor told me I had preeclampsia, that this is common for Black women, and I should have paid more attention." Fortunately, her little boy did well.

Two years later Tony became pregnant again. Although she enjoyed her first pregnancy, even with an untimely birth, she and Darren were afraid. She said, "I'm terrified it will happen again!"

She continued, "Originally we wanted to have three kids, and we are, but I just didn't expect it to be like this." Tony was pregnant with twins. On ultrasound, one of the twins was notably smaller than the other. This second pregnancy was difficult emotionally and physically. Again, Tony had hypertension in pregnancy and then developed mild cardiomyopathy. At first, she attributed fatigue, shortness of breath, and swollen ankles to being pregnant with twins. Her doctor explained to her that there is a link between the preeclampsia with her first pregnancy and the development of her cardiomyopathy (see Bello, Rendon, & Arany, 2013; Irizarry et al., 2017).

She hoped her cardiomyopathy would not worsen so she could be healthy enough to raise three children. She knew her condition was serious. She realized both she and her little boy could have died during the first pregnancy. With the subsequent development of cardiomyopathy in the second pregnancy, her fear was palpable. She considered having a tubal ligation with her planned cesarean birth, even if the second twin did not survive. She worried if this was the right decision, how her husband was doing, but mostly she worried about her *broken heart*.

The Life Course of Four Childbearing Women

These stories are the lived experiences, the unfolding of the life courses, of four mothers. Their stories are forever embedded in their memories (see Table 3.1).

TABLE 3.1 Using Life Course Theory to Examine the Lived Experiences of Four Mothers

THE MOTHER	THE STORY	TRAJECTORY AND TRANSITION	THE TURNING POINT	THE OUTCOME
Emma	No time to Lose	Emma's pregnancy was unexpected but congruent with her life trajectory. She was transitioning seamlessly to being a mother of four when she experienced severe maternal morbidity.	The two prior cesarean births increased risk for placenta previa. The vaginal exam by an unsupervised medical student when she was bleeding was a huge error compounding the existing hemorrhage.	Emma had a life-threatening hemorrhage that progressed to DIC. In other less isolated circumstances, her placenta previa would have been diagnosed early. She would have been monitored carefully and possibly had a scheduled cesarean before hemorrhage or had a faster turnaround on cesarean with immediate in-house staff available. Immediate NICU services would have been available and Brandon would have been in the barn with his Dad, feeding the calves.
Jenny	Ghosts of the Past	Jenny attempted to chart the trajectory of her life but the transition to motherhood derailed her life plans.	The birth of her daughter changed the dynamics of her marriage and the trajectory of her life. It was at this point that she began to experience severe mental illness symptoms.	Jenny sought to overcome her past adversities but mental illness was a barrier. Her lived experience of childbearing affected the dynamics in her family and charted the trajectory of her life.

(continued)

TABLE 3.1 Using Life Course Theory to Examine the Lived Experiences of Four Mothers (*continued*)

THE MOTHER	THE STORY	TRAJECTORY AND TRANSITION	THE TURNING POINT	THE OUTCOME
Sarah	A New Beginning	Sarah was on a professional trajectory, as she had planned, but longed for a child. When she became pregnant, this transition brought the problems in her marriage sharply to the forefront.	Tom's insistence on an abortion and Sarah's refusal was the turning point in their relationship. This was the first time she refused to capitulate to his wishes. His anger manifested itself in verbal and physical abuse.	To escape the control of her abusive partner, Sarah chose to be a single mother. Fortunately, she was well educated and able to return to her former employment. Tom's mother continued to be a support over the years, even as Tom went on to develop new relationships. Tom never developed a relationship with his child and had two subsequent marriages ending in divorce, both with restraining orders due to intimate partner violence. His alcoholism escalated and he was a near miss for suicide before entering alcohol rehabilitation.
Tony	A Broken Heart	Allopathic stress, racism, limited support and information at the transition of entering motherhood	Preeclampsia with the first pregnancy	Tony had a cesarean birth with the twins at 37 weeks as the second twin was not growing. They were fraternal, a boy and a girl. The girl always remained smaller. The family thrived but Tony had a damaged heart and had to remain under medical care for the remainder of her life. She decided to have a tubal ligation after the birth of the twins.

DIC, disseminating intravascular coagulation; NICU, neonatal intensive care unit.

Throughout their lives, and especially in their later years, women reminisce about these powerful events, the people who supported them, those who did not, and the turning points that shaped the trajectories of their lives.

SUMMARY

Every woman's childbearing journey is uniquely informed by prior life experiences, and the journey itself becomes a part of her very being. Prior health and life experiences factor greatly into maternal health. Healthcare providers familiar with life course theory can identify critical social determinants potentially affecting maternal health and use this important data for care. Life course theory provides a holistic framework for understanding and meeting a mother's needs and desires for her childbearing journey, whether it is her first journey into motherhood or a road previously traveled.

WHAT IF

This section poses critical questions about life course theory as it pertains to America's maternal health crisis. It is an opportunity to think about the effects of prior life and health experiences on maternal morbidity and mortality. The solutions to this national epidemic lie in interdisciplinary, imaginative conversation and problem solving. The authors invite the readers to consider these questions and add additional ones.

THE LIVED EXPERIENCE OF CHILDBEARING: THE LIFELONG IMPACT

Under what circumstances can utilization of life course theory best serve childbearing women?

How can understanding prior life experiences improve maternal health outcomes?

What could have changed the trajectory, transition, and turning point for each of the four mothers in the examples?

What can healthcare professionals do to mitigate the impact of negative childbearing experiences and outcomes?

REFERENCES

Allen, D., Feinberg, E., & Mitchell, H. (2014). Bringing life course home: A pilot to reduce pregnancy risk through housing access and family support. *Maternal and Child Health Journal, 18*(2), 405–412. doi:10.1007/s10995-013-1327-5

Alwin, D. (2012). Integrating varieties of life course concepts. *The Journals of Gerontology, Series B: Psychological Sciences and Social Sciences, 67*(2), 206–220. doi:10.1093/geronb/gbr146

Bello, N., Rendon, I., & Arany, Z. (2013). The relationship between pre-eclampsia and peripartum cardiomyopathy: A systematic review and meta-analysis. *Journal of the American College of Cardiology, 62*(18), 1715–1723. doi:10.1016/j.jacc.2013.08.717

Bermele, C., Andresen, P., & Urbanski, S. (2018). Educating nurses to screen and intervene for intimate partner violence during pregnancy. *Nursing for Women's Health, 22*(1), 79–86. doi:10.1016/j.nwh.2017.12.006

Bianchi, A. L. (2016). Intimate partner violence during the childbearing years. *Journal of Obstetric, Gynecologic & Neonatal Nursing, 45*(4), 577–578. doi:10.1016/j.jogn.2016.03.140

Birch Petersen, K., Sylvest, R., Nyboe Andersen, A., Pinborg, A., Westring Hvidman, H., & Schmidt, L. (2016). Attitudes towards family formation in cohabiting and single childless women in their mid- to late thirties. *Human Fertility, 19*(1), 48–55. doi:10.3109/14647273.2016.1156171

Black, B. P., Holditch-Davis, D., & Miles, M. S. (2009). Life course theory as a framework to examine becoming a mother of a medically fragile preterm infant. *Research in Nursing & Health, 32*(1), 38–49. doi:10.1002/nur.20298

Building U.S. Capacity to Review and Prevent Maternal Deaths. (2018). *Report from nine maternal mortality review committees*. Retrieved from http://reviewtoaction.org/Report_from_Nine_MMRCs

Centers for Disease Control and Prevention. (n.d.). PRAMS. Retrieved from https://www.cdc.gov/prams/index.htm

Cheng, T., & Solomon, B. (2014). Translating Life Course theory to clinical practice to address health disparities. *Maternal and Child Health Journal, 18*(2), 389–395. doi:10.1007/s10995-013-1279-9

Fine, A., & Kotelchuck, M. (2010). *Rethinking MCH: The life course model as an organizing framework*. Rockville, MD: U.S. Department of Health and Human Services. Retrieved from https://www.hrsa.gov/sites/default/files/ourstories/mchb75th/images/rethinkingmch.pdf

Geronimus, A., Hicken, M., Keene, D., & Bound, J. (2006). "Weathering" and age patterns of allostatic load scores among Blacks and Whites in the United States. *American Journal of Public Health, 96*(5), 826–833. doi:10.2105/AJPH.2004.060749

Halfon, N., & Hochstein, M. (2002). Life course health development: An integrated framework for developing health, policy, and research. *Milbank Quarterly, 80*(3), 433–479. doi:10.1111/1468-0009.00019

Halfon, N., Larson, K., Lu, M., Tullis, E., & Russ, S. (2014). Lifecourse health development: Past, present, and future. *Maternal and Child Health Journal, 18*(2), 344–365. doi:10.1007/s10995-013-1346-2

Hutchison, M., & Thomas, M. (2017). Circles of change: CenteringPregnancy®, health disparities, and vulnerable women. In B. Anderson, J. Rooks, & R. Barroso (Eds.), *Best practices in midwifery: Using the evidence to implement change* (2nd ed., pp. 199–215). New York, NY: Springer Publishing Company.

Irizarry, O., Levine, L., Lewey, J., Boyer, T., Riis, V., Elovitz, M., & Arany, Z. (2017). Comparison of clinical characteristics and outcomes of peripartum cardiomyopathy between African American and non–African American women. *JAMA Cardiology, 2*(11), 1256–1260. doi:10.1001/jamacardio.2017.3574

Isenberg, N. (2017). *White trash: The 400-year untold history of class in America*. New York, NY: Penguin Books.

King, T., & Pinger, W. (2014). Evidence-based practice for intrapartum care: The pearls of midwifery. *Journal of Midwifery and Women's Health, 59*(6), 572–585. doi:10.1111/jmwh.12261

Kothari, C., Liepman, M., Tareen, R., Florian, P., Charoth, R., Haas, S., . . . Curtis, A. (2016). Intimate partner violence associated with postpartum depression, regardless of socioeconomic status. *Maternal and Child Health Journal, 20*(6), 1237–1246. doi:10.1007/s10995-016-1925-0

Loftman, P. (2017). Racial and ethnic disparities in birth outcomes: The challenge to midwifery. In B. Anderson, J. Rooks, & R. Barroso (Eds.), *Best practices in midwifery: Using the evidence to implement change* (2nd ed., 183–198). New York, NY: Springer Publishing Company.

Miesnik, S., & Stringer, M. (2002). Technology in the birthing room. *Nursing Clinics of North America, 37*(4), 781–793. doi:10.1016/S0029-6465(02)00025-7

Mortimer, J., & Shanahan, M. (Eds.). (2003). *Handbook of the life course* (3rd ed.). New York, NY: Springer.

Orsolini, L., Valchera, A., Vecchiotti, R., Tomasetti, C., Iasevoli, F., Fornaro, M., . . . Bellantuono, C. (2016). Suicide during perinatal period: Epidemiology, risk factors, and clinical correlates. *Frontiers in Psychiatry, 7*, 138. doi:10.3389/fpsyt.2016.00138

Owens, T., & Jackson, F. M. (2015). Examining life-course socioeconomic position, contextualized stress, and depression among well-educated African-American pregnant women. *Women's Health Issues, 25*(4), 382–389. doi:10.1016/j.whi.2015.05.001

Peck, E. (2018, May 27). Everyone is missing a key reason the U.S. birth rate is declining. *Huffington Post*. Retrieved from https://www.huffingtonpost.com/entry/key-reason-birth-rate-declining_us_5b0725cfe4b0568a88097feb

Simoni, M., Mu, L., & Collins, S. (2017). Women's career priority is associated with attitudes towards family planning and ethical acceptance of reproductive technologies. *Human Reproduction, 32*(10), 2069–2075. doi:10.1093/humrep/dex275

Sockol, L., & Battle, C. (2015). Maternal attitudes, depression, and anxiety in pregnant and postpartum multiparous women. *Archives of Women's Mental Health, 18*(4), 585–593. doi:10.1007/s00737-015-0511-6

United Nations Human Rights Council. (2018). *Report of the Special Rapporteur on extreme poverty and human rights on his mission to the United States of America*. Retrieved from https://digitallibrary.un.org/record/1629536/files/A_HRC_38_33_Add-1-EN.pdf

United Nations Population Fund. (2012). *Rich mother, poor mother: The social determinants of maternal death and disability*. Retrieved from https://www.unfpa.org/sites/default/files/resource-pdf/EN-SRH%20fact%20sheet-Poormother.pdf

Wadhwa, P., Garite, T., Porto, M., Glynn, L., Chicz-DeMet, A., Dunkel-Schetter, C., & Sandman, C. A. (2004). Placental corticotropin-releasing hormone (CRH), spontaneous preterm birth, and fetal growth restriction: A prospective investigation. *American Journal of Obstetrics and Gynecology, 191*(4), 1063–1069. doi:10.1016/j.ajog.2004.06.070

Woolf, S., & Aron, L. (Eds.). (2013). *U.S. health in international perspective: Shorter lives, poorer health*. Washington, DC: National Academies Press.

World Health Organization. (n.d.-a). Child and adolescent health. Retrieved from http://www.euro.who.int/en/health-topics/Life-stages/child-and-adolescent-health/child-and-adolescent-health

World Health Organization. (n.d.-b). Maternal and newborn health. Retrieved from http://www.euro.who.int/en/health-topics/Life-stages/maternal-and-newborn-health/maternal-and-newborn-health

Wyoming Department of Health. (n.d.). Pregnancy Risk Assessment Monitoring System (PRAMS). Retrieved from https://health.wyo.gov/publichealth/chronic-disease-and-maternal-child-health-epidemiology-unit/mch-epi/pregnancy-risk-assessment-monitoring-system-prams

THE HEALTHCARE DELIVERY SYSTEM

Structural Challenges

EILEEN K. FRY-BOWERS

OBJECTIVES

At the end of this chapter, the reader will be able to:

1. Describe the healthcare delivery system and insurance systems in the United States.
2. Discuss policies, laws, and institutional mandates that impact maternal health.
3. Identify key steps needed for reform of the healthcare system.

THE HEALTHCARE SYSTEM IN THE UNITED STATES

One tragic shortcoming is the rising rate of maternal death and severe maternal morbidity in the United States. Many mothers do not die at the time of giving birth but rather in the 1st year postpartum (Creanga, Syverson, Seed, & Callaghan, 2017). In addition, mortality rates are rising for all women of reproductive age, not just those who are bearing children (Declercq & Shah, 2018). This chapter addresses the structural characteristics of the U.S. health system that impact the care of women of reproductive age with focus on care during the perinatal and extended postpartum periods. Quality improvement initiatives, including the use of evidence-based toolkits and safety bundles that standardize care and reduce risk, are discussed in subsequent chapters. This chapter focuses on the scope of public and private insurance in providing access to care, the impact of public and institutional policy, and the key steps toward healthcare reform in the United States.

The term "industrialized nation" refers to the 36-member Organisation for Economic Co-Operation and Development (OECD) of which the United States is a member (OECD, 2018). Unlike most industrialized nations in OECD, the United States does not operate a national health service, offer a single-payer national health insurance system, or manage a multipayer universal health insurance fund. The United States lacks a uniform health system and does not guarantee universal access to care. At best, it can be described as a multitiered hybrid quasi-system dependent on private and public financing.

In 2016, health spending in the United States was $10,348 per person, more than 30% higher than Switzerland, the next highest per capita spender. U.S. public expenditures on health, about 8.5% of the gross domestic product (GDP), are comparable to other industrialized countries that publicly finance their entire health systems (OECD, 2014). In addition, U.S. private spending (8.8% GDP) far exceeds the average among those nations (Sawyer & Cox, 2018). Greater overall U.S. spending (17.3% GDP public and private combined) is likely driven by higher healthcare prices and use of technology rather than increased utilization of provider visits or hospitalizations. Conversely, U.S. spending on social support services, for example, housing assistance, employment programs, food security, and retirement and disability benefits, comprises a much smaller share of the economy compared to other countries (Squires, 2015). In a 10-year analysis of national-level health and social service spending and health outcome data from the OECD, the United States had the lowest ratio of social service spending compared to healthcare spending (Bradley, Sipsma, & Taylor, 2017). On average, countries with lower ratios of social service spending fare worse than counterparts with higher social service spending. It is not surprising then that Americans have poorer health outcomes, including shorter life expectancy, and greater prevalence of chronic conditions compared to international peers (Bradley et al., 2017; Squires, 2015). This health disparity is most apparent among socioeconomically disadvantaged groups. However, the National Academy of Medicine reports that poorer health in the United States is not just the result of economic, social, or racial and ethnic disadvantages. Advantaged, nonsmoking, nonobese Americans also experience worse health than their counterparts in other countries (Woolf & Aron, 2013).

The role that the U.S. healthcare system plays in these disparities is a subject of debate. Current outcome measures may not be fully explained by gaps in insurance or access to or coordination of care (Woolf & Aron, 2013). In comparing the U.S. public health and medical care systems to those of other countries, lack of consistent and analogous data prevents comparison with other nations (Woolf & Aron, 2013). Woolf and Aron (2013) state, "Conditions that are treatable by health care have many origins, and causal factors outside the clinic may matter as much as the benefits or limitations of medical care" (p. 134). Health outcomes may not simply relate to contemporary U.S. health system performance but also to the social determinants of health. Substantial evidence supports the notion that early life course, which encompasses genetic, biological, behavioral, social, and economic determinants, has implications for health years or decades later (Halfon & Hochstein, 2002; Halfon, Larson, Lu, Tullis, & Russ, 2014). When and where an individual grew up and the social and economic conditions of the family are likely to impact health status across the life span regardless of health system utilization. Regardless of social and economic conditions, collective data reveal that the current U.S. public health and healthcare systems have important shortcomings (Woolf & Aron, 2013).

ACCESS TO CARE: THE ROLE OF HEALTH INSURANCE

Most OECD countries and other developed nations mandate universal healthcare coverage and provide access to care by utilizing one of three types of health insurance programs: a national health service, a national health insurance system, or a multipayer (all payer) health insurance system (Table 4.1).

Conversely, the United States relies on a hybrid system of publicly and privately financed health insurance that developed over the course of the 20th century, as much by historical circumstance as by design (Toland, 2014). As a result, coverage gaps exist and many women lack access to care throughout their reproductive years.

Private Insurance

Employer-Sponsored Insurance

Employer-sponsored insurance (ESI) is the largest single source of health insurance for Americans. About half of all nonelderly Americans are covered by an employer-sponsored plan (either as employees or as dependents). Also known as "group health insurance," this coverage may be fully subsidized by the employer or the employee may contribute to the expense via monthly payments (premiums), copayments, or deductibles (also known as "cost sharing"; Kaiser Family

TABLE 4.1 Most Frequent Types of Healthcare Coverage in OECD Countries

TYPE OF COVERAGE	DESCRIPTION
National health service	Healthcare is provided and financed by the government
National health insurance system	Single-payer government-run insurance program that every citizen pays into; pays out all healthcare costs; no profit motive; uses private sector providers; has considerable market power to lower prices
Multipayer health insurance system	Sickness funds, financed jointly by employers and employees through payroll taxes; no profit motive; government maintains significant cost control

OECD, Organisation for Economic Co-operation and Development.

Foundation, 2017b). Choices and cost of coverage often depend upon the size of the company with smaller companies offering fewer and often more costly options.

The number of Americans who have ESI has been declining. In 1999, 67% of nonelderly workers were covered by ESI. By 2014, 56% were covered. This decline in coverage is most pronounced among workers with low to modest income (Long, Rae, Claxton, & Damico, 2016). For those still eligible for ESI, quality of coverage has declined (Blumenthal, 2017). In 2016 nearly 25% of working-age adults eligible for ESI had such high out-of-pocket costs and deductibles relative to their income that they were effectively underinsured (Collins, Gunja, & Doty, 2017).

Individual Private Insurance

Individuals without access to ESI may purchase "nongroup" or individual plans for themselves or their families through a private insurance company. Historically, pricing and options varied substantially by health history and by state or county of residence. Companies could deny or rescind coverage based upon preexisting health conditions. Few companies covered maternity care or required additional premiums to provide such coverage. As a result, many families of reproductive age were unable to obtain health insurance coverage during childbearing.

Public Policy to Prevent Insurance Discrimination During Childbearing

The Pregnancy Discrimination Act of 1978 is an amendment to Title VII of the 1964 Civil Rights Act. It is a federal statute that prohibits discrimination based on gender, childbearing, or pregnancy-related conditions. It requires ESI plans offered by employers with 15 or more employees to cover pregnancy, childbirth, and pregnancy-related conditions similar to temporarily disabling conditions (Pregnancy Discrimination Act, 1978). Since 1978 nearly all ESI group health plans have provided coverage for childbearing (Kaiser Family Foundation, 2010).

The Health Insurance Portability and Accountability Act (HIPAA) of 1996 effectively extended this coverage to small employer groups (defined as companies with 2–50 employees; HIPAA, 1996; Kaiser Family Foundation, 2010). Prior to the 2010 signing and implementation of the Patient Protection and Affordable Care Act (ACA, 2010), 75% of these health plans did not cover inpatient maternity care, including the birth (Kaiser Family Foundation, 2010). In addition, only 12 states required individual or nongroup plans to cover childbearing. Four of these states required such coverage only in health maintenance organization (HMO) plans, usually with additional premium costs and annual limits as low as $2,000. For women covered by private insurance, the average cost of pregnancy care and delivery is more than $32,000 for a vaginal birth and $51,000 for a cesarean section without complications (Palanker, Volk, & Giovannelli, 2017).

On March 23, 2010, President Barack Obama signed into law the ACA. The law requires individual and small group plans without a "grandfather" clause to cover essential health benefits (EHB; Centers for Medicare and Medicaid Services

[CMS], n.d.). Individual health insurance policies purchased from insurance companies, agents, or brokers on or before March 23, 2010, are exempted from certain provisions of the ACA and may not include some rights and protections. Plans can lose their grandfather status if they make significant changes that reduce benefits or increase costs to consumers (HealthCare.gov, n.d.). The ACA has had far-reaching effects, providing EHB for the following categories of care:

- Ambulatory patient services
- Emergency services
- Hospitalization
- Maternity and newborn care
- Mental health and substance use disorder treatment including behavioral health treatment
- Prescription drugs
- Rehabilitative and habilitative services and devices
- Laboratory services
- Preventive/wellness services and chronic disease management
- Pediatric services, including oral and vision care (CMS, n.d.)

The ACA prevents insurance companies from denying or rescinding coverage (unless fraud is proven) or charging customers a surcharge based upon health status. It eliminates limits or lifetime caps on individual coverage. For those who must purchase insurance outside of ESI or group-sponsored environments, it creates new marketplaces or exchanges for the sale of plans by private insurance companies. Low-income individuals and families purchasing insurance through the marketplace or exchange may qualify for subsidized coverage. From 2010 through 2015, as a result of the ACA individual mandate, which required individuals to demonstrate proof of coverage, an estimated 19.2 million nonelderly people gained health insurance coverage, including approximately 5 million women of childbearing age (19–44 years old). Under the ACA, every U.S. state realized overall increased insurance coverage (Garrett & Gangopadhyaya, 2016).

Even though the ACA has increased insurance for maternity care, some women still lack access to coverage. Presently, enrollment in ESI and individual health insurance plans takes place only during annual open enrollment periods. The only time a person can enroll outside of the open enrollment period is if they experience a "qualifying life event." Pregnancy is not a qualifying life event. Under federal rules implementing the ACA, pregnancy is covered as a "preexisting condition." The insurer cannot deny coverage if a woman is pregnant at open enrollment. To date, only New York has identified pregnancy as a qualifying life event (New York State, 2015). If a woman becomes pregnant outside of the open enrollment period and is uninsured or if she is enrolled in a grandfathered plan that does not include maternity coverage, she is barred from purchasing coverage for maternity care in the marketplace or exchange (Garro, Hern andez, & Pellegrini, 2016). Without access to maternity care coverage, she may delay care or face significant out-of-pocket costs, both of which have implications for maternal health (Garro et al., 2016).

Medicaid

Medicaid is a jointly funded, federal–state public health insurance entitlement program administered at the state level. It provides health coverage for eligible low-income U.S. residents, including pregnant women. It is the largest source of health insurance coverage for both children and adults in the nation and provides essential financial support for the nation's safety net of clinics, hospitals, and long-term care facilities (Turner, McKee, Chen & Coursolle, 2017).

Approximately two thirds of the adult women on Medicaid are between 19 and 49 years. Medicaid covers a wide range of reproductive healthcare services for these women, including family planning, testing and treatment of sexually transmitted infections, prenatal services, childbirth, and postpartum care (Kasier Family Foundation, 2017a). Medicaid is the primary source of coverage for maternity services for low-income women in the United States, financing almost 50% of all births (Markus, Krobe, Garro, Gerstein, & Pellegrini, 2017; Smith et al., 2016). Under federal law, all states participating in Medicaid must provide coverage for pregnancy-related services terminating at 60 days postpartum for women with incomes up to 138% of the federal poverty level (FPL; Gifford, Walls, Salganicoff, & Gomez, 2017). Although all states must provide some level of maternity care without cost sharing to eligible pregnant women, each state has considerable discretion on the scope of maternity care benefits. In some states, for families with modest incomes that exceed Medicaid qualification thresholds, the Children's Health Insurance Program (CHIP), a state-administered program, provides coverage for pregnant women. Coverage and eligibility requirements vary by state (Gifford et al., 2017).

Impact of the ACA on Medicaid Coverage

The ACA expands Medicaid eligibility by allowing states to extend coverage to all individuals with family incomes at or below 138% of the FPL (Gifford et al., 2017). Among those states that decided to expand Medicaid coverage with the ACA, there was a 45% overall increase in the number of all U.S. residents with health insurance compared to states that elected not to expand Medicaid (29%; Garrett & Gangopadhyaya, 2016).

In a highly publicized case in 2012, *National Federation of Independent Business v. Sebelius* (2012), the U.S. Supreme Court ruled that Medicaid expansion under the ACA is an optional decision for states. The result is inconsistent coverage across the country. As of February 2019, 36 states and the District of Columbia (DC) have adopted Medicaid expansion (Kaiser Family Foundation, 2019). In these states, the expansion program extends coverage for new mothers beyond the 60-day postpartum period (Gifford et al., 2017). Three more states are presently considering expansion and 14 states have decided not to expand coverage (Kaiser Family Foundation, 2018a). However, most states, even those that have not expanded Medicaid to the general low-income adult population, offer coverage to pregnant women at the federal minimum threshold of 138% FPL through Medicaid/CHIP (Gifford et al., 2017).

As of early 2018, 17 states provide Medicaid coverage for pregnant women with incomes of 138% up to 200% FPL; 22 states cover pregnant women with incomes of 200% to 250% FPL; 12 states, including DC, cover pregnant women with family incomes above 250% FPL. Through CHIP funding, 16 states provide coverage through the "unborn child option," defining an unborn child as existing from conception to birth. This allows states to cover income-eligible pregnant women regardless of legal immigration status (Kaiser Family Foundation, 2018). In states without Medicaid expansion with ACA, women in general can qualify for coverage only if they belong to an eligible group, that is, pregnant, parent with dependent children, senior, or disabled, and meet the state-specific income criteria, which range from 18% FPL in Alabama and Texas to 105% FPL in Maine. This restriction means that a woman may not have ongoing healthcare and management of chronic illness prior to becoming pregnant or between pregnancies (Kasier Family Foundation, 2017a). In states without Medicaid expansion, she loses coverage at 60 days postpartum, although she may qualify for decreased Medicaid assistance as the parent of a dependent child. The income threshold for this category is typically much lower than during pregnancy and may even disqualify her (Gifford et al., 2017).

Medicare

Medicare is a federally financed, federally administered health insurance program that serves most individuals over the age of 65 years, younger individuals with disabilities, and persons with end-stage renal disease. While not usually associated with childbearing, Medicare does provide maternity care coverage for women with Social Security disability benefits. Women in this category are responsible for the hospital deductible fee and any cost-sharing payments associated with outpatient services. Low-income pregnant women in Medicare may also qualify for Medicaid. The coverage varies by state. Because Medicare coverage is determined by age or disability status, coverage continues following the birth of the child (Barry, 2009).

NARROWED NETWORKS FOR MATERNAL CARE
Provider Networks

A provider network is the group of doctors, other healthcare providers, and hospitals with whom an insurance plan has a contract. Generally, these providers are called "network providers" or "in-network providers," and a provider that is not contracted with the insurance plan is referred to as an "out-of-network provider." Typically, the in-network provider delivers care at a lower cost to the patient compared to seeking care from an out-of-network provider (CMS, 2017). As healthcare costs rise and as the ACA marketplaces evolve, narrow provider networks have become a controversial source of potential savings for both the individual and group (ESI) insurance markets. Evidence regarding reducing cost versus risk of reducing access and quality of care is mixed (Blake, 2015; Dafny, Hendel, Marone, & Ody, 2017; Polsky, Cidav, & Swanson, 2016; Spurlock & Shannon, 2015). These networks have the potential to reduce a woman's choice for maternal care providers and sites of care.

Narrowed Networks: An Exemplar

Narrowed networks become an important consideration when examining the relationship between faith-based institutions and the provision of maternity care and reproductive health services. Examples of impact are ethical choices about regular and emergency contraception, tubal ligation, abortion, infertility, sexually transmitted infections, ectopic pregnancy, culturally responsive care regardless of sexual orientation, do-not-resuscitate choices for both mothers and babies, and saving the life of the mother or the baby preferentially. There are limited maternal health outcome studies investigating these conflicts as well as discrepancies between evidence-based, legally sanctioned care and provider stance or institutional policy on these ethical issues.

One in six hospital beds (American Civil Liberties Union [ACLU], 2016) and four out of the top five largest not-for-profit health systems in the United States are Roman Catholic owned or affiliated (Bricker, n.d.). The number of owned or affiliated hospitals varies by region. For example, Catholic health systems are quite prevalent in the Midwest and more than 40% of hospital beds in Washington state are Catholic affiliated. In many rural communities, the only hospital is a Catholic facility (Kaye, Amiri, Melling, & Dalven, 2016), and for some women, this facility may be their only in-network provider. This narrow network affects both private- and Medicaid-managed care plans, potentially restricting choices of maternity and reproductive care services and providers.

Catholic facilities have historically played a significant role in the nation's healthcare and the public health safety net in many positive ways supportive to family growth and development. However, the expansion of Catholic healthcare systems has disproportionately impacted legal reproductive healthcare choices, especially for low-income women in many communities (Shepherd, Platt, Franke, & Boylan, 2017). Women may not understand that reproductive health services and choices about maternity care may be restricted and providers are not under obligation to inform women of this fact (Sawicki, 2016).

The Ethical and Religious Directives for Catholic Health Care is a set of 77 directives governing the care that Catholic hospitals provide, regardless of the religious beliefs of the patient seeking services or the healthcare provider delivering services

(U.S. Conference of Catholic Bishops, 2018). A woman receiving care at a Catholic facility is under the following directives:

- Antiovulatory medication may be provided in cases of sexual assault when it can be proven that pregnancy has not occurred (Directive 36)

- No abortion, including for cases of rape or incest (Directive 45)

- No contraception, except for natural family planning (Directive 52)

- No treatment for ectopic pregnancy (Directive 48)

- No sterilization (Directive 53; U.S. Conference of Catholic Bishops, 1018)

Another directive, Directive 46, speaks to severe maternal morbidity. This directive states, "Operations, treatments, and medications that have as their direct purpose the cure of a proportionately serious pathological condition of a pregnant woman are permitted when they cannot be safely postponed until the unborn child is viable, even if they will result in the death of the unborn child" (U.S. Conference of Catholic Bishops, 2018, p. 19). However, the local bishop, not the physician, is the authoritative interpreter of all directives. As a result, some facilities practice a no-terminations-ever policy, leaving no options for women in life-threatening situations. This interpretation extends to approval of referrals for women to receive prohibited care elsewhere. In a recent study, OB/GYN physicians in Catholic facilities reported that administrators and ethicists demonstrated attitudes and practices about referrals ranging from encouragement and tolerance to active discouragement (Stulberg, Jackson, & Freedman, 2016). In some cases, physicians kept referrals hidden. The physicians stated that referrals were not always sufficient to meet the needs of low-income patients or timely in those with urgent medical conditions (Stulberg et al., 2016). The standard of care provided to women by Catholic hospitals can vary, ranging from excellence to deviance from evidence-based best practice.

The American College of Obstetricians and Gynecologists (ACOG) takes issue with a provider exerting control over legal reproductive services. In regard to health provider refusal to perform certain procedures, the Committee on Ethics of the ACOG states "refusals should be limited if they constitute an imposition of religious or moral beliefs on patients, negatively affect a patient's health, are based on scientific misinformation, or create or reinforce racial or socioeconomic inequalities. Conscientious refusals that conflict with patient well-being should be accommodated only if the primary duty to the patient can be fulfilled" (ACOG, 2007, para. 1).

Challenges to the ACA

Taken as a whole, the ACA has been one of the most controversial legislative issues of our time. *New York Times* columnist and Princeton University economist Paul Krugman declared in a *Times* article on January 13, 2011, that the debate over healthcare reform can be viewed as a tale of two moralities shaped by two worldviews. He stated, "One side saw health reform . . . as fulfilling a moral imperative. . . . The other side saw the same reform as a moral outrage, an assault on the right of Americans to spend their money as they choose" (Krugman, 2011, p. 7). One of the most contentious aspects of the ACA is Medicaid expansion to cover childbearing women. Opponents arguing against Medicaid-expanded coverage state that men and postmenopausal women do not need maternity coverage and should not be required to pay for it through taxation. Harvard economist Greg Mankiw argued, "Having children is more a choice than a random act of nature. People who drive a new Porsche pay more for car insurance than those who drive an old Chevy. . . . Why isn't having children viewed in the same way?" (Franke-Ruta, 2013, p. 3).

Setting aside the fact that nearly half of all pregnancies in the United States each year are unintended (Finer & Zolna, 2016), this view does not incorporate the concept of pooled risk in insurance, nor does it address the lasting benefits of healthy mothers and children to society at large (Palanker, Volk, & Giovannelli, 2017; Sonfield, 2017). It also does not answer the question of whether a young, employed mother should be required to contribute, for example, to the pooled insurance care of an elderly man with prostate cancer.

Why did supporting motherhood become controversial? One answer is that the opposition to this coverage is not rooted in the coverage itself or in the argument about pooled risk. Rather it is rooted in discrimination and racism. Because a significant number of women, especially married women, have ESI, which is required to cover maternity care, the coverage mandated through the ACA has its greatest impact on unmarried women, women of low to moderate income, and women of color (Franke-Ruta, 2013).

Since its passage, over 100 federal lawsuits have been filed against the ACA, two of which were adjudicated by the U.S. Supreme Court. The U.S. House of Representatives has voted on at least 62 measures to repeal or defund the ACA. Public opinion, as well as empirical evidence of impact, remains mixed and is substantially influenced by age, race, political affiliation, health and employment status, educational level, and geographical region. With a unified government (a Republican president and Republican-controlled Congress), major changes in healthcare and unraveling of the public health safety net have occurred. More changes are anticipated. Although initial legislative attempts to repeal the ACA failed, if passed, these bills would undo some of the ACA's most important protections for maternal and reproductive health.

Access to preventive care and other reproductive services, including contraceptives, chronic disease screenings and treatment, and sexually transmitted infection testing and treatment, would be significantly curtailed. In addition, drastic cuts to Medicaid and an end to the Medicaid expansion would negatively impact access to maternity care, especially among low-income women and poor women of color. Finally, these bills would undermine the EHB requirement, rendering coverage for maternity care once again out of reach for many women of childbearing age

(Gamble & Taylor, 2017). Erosion of coverage is occurring and government actions to increase the availability of insurance policies that do not comply with ACA's minimum EHB standards continue to threaten access to care (Collins, Gunja, Doty, & Bhupal, 2018).

REFORM OF THE HEALTHCARE SYSTEM

The challenge of rising maternal morbidity and mortality in the United States requires changes in public policy and aggressive system reform of both public and private-sector health systems. Comprehensive reproductive healthcare must be integrated into ongoing payment and delivery system reform. Specifically, national provider and advocacy groups have developed a set of priorities organized around five core areas with the goals of improving reproductive healthcare and outcomes as well as lowering costs (Sonfield, 2016):

- *Access to care.* Women should have access to the full range of reproductive health services and be able to choose, without interference, specific evidence-based reproductive health services that best meet their needs.

- *Access to providers.* Women should have unimpeded direct access to a comprehensive choice of providers without referral for maternity and gynecologic care.

- *Patient safeguards.* Reform initiatives should include an array of patient protections, including but not limited to choices among providers; clear information, especially about the scope and quality of care offered by providers; access to all covered services without barriers and free from ideologic interference; access to and control over their health information and records; and access to coverage and culturally competent trauma-informed care regardless of language or literacy.

- *Payments and investments.* Providers should be fully reimbursed for the services offered and should account for the value of preventing unintended pregnancies, sexually transmitted infections, and reproductive cancers, and any financial incentives should promote quality improvement and address reproductive health needs and disparities.

- *Patient and provider engagement.* Representatives of the patient and provider communities should collaborate to ensure that care is actually meeting the needs of the population served (Sonfield, 2016).

While not devised to address the particular issue of maternal morbidity and mortality, these public policy principles would improve the quality of reproductive health services more broadly, a necessary precursor to solving the current maternal health crisis. Beyond payment and delivery system reform, public health reform should also include the establishment and consistent use of state-level multidisciplinary committees (e.g., maternal mortality and severe maternal morbidity review boards) to track, analyze, and identify locally relevant solutions to prevent maternal deaths and severe morbidity. In addition, recognizing that significant risk factors for maternal mortality and morbidity exist outside of the healthcare delivery system supports measures to address substance use, delay in prenatal risk assessment, lack of social support, food and housing insecurity, mental health problems, family violence or neglect, and environmental or occupational hazards.

SUMMARY

Economic factors can present a barrier to accessing appropriate and timely maternal healthcare. The availability of affordable public or private insurance is key to ensuring that childbearing women receive essential services. Adequate insurance coverage increases the likelihood of women receiving preventive services and management of chronic conditions pre- and inter-conceptually. While access to health insurance does not, in itself, eliminate disparities and the social determinants of health, it is supportive to healthier childbearing. A concerted effort to mend the porous public health safety net is absolutely essential.

WHAT IF

This section poses critical questions about how the healthcare system in the United States contributes to the crippling of health and the loss of life among America's mothers. It is an opportunity to think about the effects of health policy and access to care. The solutions to this national epidemic lie in interdisciplinary, imaginative conversation and problem solving. The authors invite the readers to consider these questions and add more.

THE HEALTHCARE DELIVERY SYSTEM: STRUCTURAL CHALLENGES

Discuss the historical emergence of the current healthcare system in America.

How do the current healthcare delivery and insurance systems improve or contribute to the maternal health crisis in America?

Describe legislation that has protected or undermined maternal health.

Who are the players in addressing healthcare reform? How does each player contribute to the discussion about healthcare reform?

How would maternal health be impacted if the United States went to a single-payer healthcare system?

REFERENCES

American Civil Liberities Union. (2016). *New report reveals 1 in 6 U.S. hospital beds are in Catholic facilities that prohibit essential health care for women* [Press release]. Retrieved from https://www.aclu.org/news/new-report-reveals-1-6-us-hospital-beds-are-catholic-facilities-prohibit-essential-health-care

American College of Obstetricians and Gynecologists. (2007). ACOG Committee Opinion No. 385: The limits of conscientious refusal in reproductive medicine (reaffirmed 2016). Retrieved from https://www.acog.org/Clinical-Guidance-and-Publications/Committee-Opinions/Committee-on-Ethics/The-Limits-of-Conscientious-Refusal-in-Reproductive-Medicine

Barry, P. (2009). Does Medicare cover pregnancy? *AARP Bulletin.* Retrieved from https://www.aarp.org/health/medicare-insurance/info-05-2009/ask_ms_medicare_question_57_.html

Blake, V. (2015). Narrow networks, the very sick, and the Patient Protection and Affordable Care Act: Recalling the purpose of health insurance and reform. *Minnesota Journal of Law, Science & Technology, 16*(1), Article 4. Available at https://scholarship.law.umn.edu/mjlst/vol16/iss1/4

Blumenthal, D. (2017). The decline of employer-sponsored health insurance. Retrieved from https://www.commonwealthfund.org/blog/2017/decline-employer-sponsored-health-insurance

Bradley, E., Sipsma, H., & Taylor, L. (2017). American health care paradox—High spending on health care and poor health. *QJM: An International Journal of Medicine, 110*(2), 61–65. doi:10.1093/qjmed/hcw187

Bricker, E. (n.d.). Healthcare fast facts—Top 30 largest hospital systems in America. Retrieved from https://ideas.alight.com/health/healthcare-fast-facts-top-30-largest-hospital-systems-in-america

Centers for Medicare and Medicaid Services. (n.d.). Information on essential health benefits (EHB) benchmark plans. Retrieved from https://www.cms.gov/cciio/resources/data-resources/ehb.html

Centers for Medicare and Medicaid Services. (2017). *What you should know about provider networks* (CMS Product No. 11766). Retrieved from https://marketplace.cms.gov/outreach-and-education/what-you-should-know-provider-networks.pdf

Collins, S., Gunja, M., & Doty, M. (2017). How well does insurance coverage protect consumers from health care costs? Retrieved from https://www.commonwealthfund.org/publications/issue-briefs/2017/oct/how-well-does-insurance-coverage-protect-consumers-health-care

Collins, S., Gunja, M., Doty, M., & Bhupal, H. (2018, May 1). First look at health insurance coverage in 2018 finds ACA gains beginning to reverse. Retrieved from https://www.commonwealthfund.org/blog/2018/first-look-health-insurance-coverage-2018-finds-aca-gains-beginning-reverse

Creanga, A., Syverson, C., Seed, K., & Callaghan, W. (2017). Pregnancy-related mortality in the United States, 2011–2013. *Obstetrics & Gynecology, 130*(2), 366–373. doi:10.1097/AOG.0000000000002114

Dafny, L., Hendel, I., Marone, V., & Ody, C. (2017). Narrow networks on the health insurance marketplaces: Prevalences, pricing, and the cost of network breadth. *Health Affairs, 36*(9), 1606–1614. doi:10.1377/hlthaff.2016.1669

Declercq, E., & Shah, N. (2018, August 22). Maternal deaths represent the canary in the coal mine for women's health. *STAT*. Retrieved from https://www.statnews.com/2018/08/22/maternal-deaths-women-health

Finer, L., & Zolna, M. (2016). Declines in unintended pregnancy in the United States, 2008–2011. *New England Journal of Medicine, 374*, 843–852. doi:10.1056/NEJMsa1506575

Franke-Ruta, G. (2013, November 22). Why is maternity care such an issue for Obamacare opponents? *The Atlantic*. Retrieved from https://www.theatlantic.com/politics/archive/2013/11/why-is-maternity-care-such-an-issue-for-obamacare-opponents/281396

Gamble, C. M., & Taylor, J. (2017). Maternity care under ACA repeal. Retrieved from https://www.americanprogress.org/issues/women/reports/2017/08/07/437116/maternity-care-aca-repeal

Garrett, B., & Gangopadhyaya, A. (2016). *Who gained health insurance coverage under the ACA, and where do they live?* Washington, DC: The Urban Institute. Retrieved from https://www.urban.org/sites/default/files/publication/86761/2001041-who-gained-health-insurance-coverage-under-the-aca-and-where-do-they-live.pdf

Garro, N., Hernandez, B., & Pellegrini, C. (2016). HHS must remove barriers to coverage for pregnant women. *Health Affairs Blog*. doi:10.1377/hblog20160219.053241

Gifford, K., Walls, J., Salganicoff, A., & Gomez, I. (2017). *Medicaid coverage of pregnancy and prenatal benefits: Results from a state survey*. Menlo Park, CA: Kaiser Family Foundation. Retrieved from http://files.kff.org/attachment/Report-Medicaid-Coverage-of-Pregnancy-and-Perinatal-Benefits

Halfon, N., & Hochstein, M. (2002). Life course health development: An integrated framework for developing health, policy, and research. *Milbank Quarterly, 80*(3), 433–479. doi:10.1111/1468-0009.00019

Halfon, N., Larson, K., Lu, M., Tullis, E., & Russ, S. (2014). Life course health development: Past, present, and future. *Maternal and Child Health Journal, 18*(2), 344–365. doi:10.1007/s10995-013-1346-2

HealthCare.gov. (n.d.). Grandfathered health plan. Retrieved from https://www.healthcare.gov/glossary/grandfathered-health-plan

Health Insurance Portability and Accountability Act, 42 U.S.C. 300gg–91 § 2791 (1996).

Ibis Reproductive Health. (2006). *Complying with the law? How Catholic hospitals respond to state laws mandating the provision of emergency contraception to sexual assault patients*. Washington, DC: Catholics for Choice. Retrieved from https://ibisreproductivehealth.org/sites/default/files/files/publications/CFC.%20Complying%20with%20the%20Law.%20February%202006.pdf

Kaiser Family Foundation. (2010). Pre-ACA state maternity coverage mandates: Individual and small group markets. Retrieved from https://www.kff.org/other/state-indicator/pre-aca-state-maternity-coverage-mandates-individual-and-small-group-markets/?currentTimeframe=0&sortModel=%7B%22colId%22:%22Location%22,%22sort%22:%22asc%22%7D

Kasier Family Foundation. (2017a). *Fact Sheet: Medicaid's role for women*. Menlo Park, CA: Author. Retrieved from http://files.kff.org/attachment/Fact-Sheet-Medicaids-Role-for-Women

Kaiser Family Foundation. (2017b). Health insurance coverage of the total population. Retrieved from https://www.kff.org/other/state-indicator/total-population/?currentTimeframe=0&sortModel=%7B%22colId%22:%22Location%22,%22sort%22:%22asc%22%7D

Kaiser Family Foundation. (2018). Where are states today? Medicaid and CHIP eligibility levels for children, pregnant women, and adults. Retrieved from https://www.kff.org/medicaid/fact-sheet/where-are-states-today-medicaid-and-chip

Kaiser Family Foundation. (2019). Status of state action on the Medicaid expansion decision. Retrieved from https://www.kff.org/health-reform/state-indicator/state-activity-around-expanding-medicaid-under-the-affordable-care-act/?currentTimeframe=0&sortModel=%7B%22colId%22:%22Location%22,%22sort%22:%22asc%22%7D

Kaye, J., Amiri, B., Melling, L., & Dalven, J. (2016). *Health care denied*. New York, NY: American Civil Liberities Union. Retrieved from https://www.aclu.org/sites/default/files/field_document/healthcaredenied.pdf

Krugman, P. (January 13, 2011). A tale of two moralities. *New York Times*. Retrieved from https://www.nytimes.com/2011/01/14/opinion/14krugman.html

Long, M., Rae, M., Claxton, G., & Damico, A. (2016). *Trends in employer-sponsored insurance offer and coverage rates, 1999–2014*. Menlo Park, CA: Kaiser Family Foundation. Retrieved from http://files.kff.org/attachment/issue-brief-trends-in-employer-sponsored-insurance-offer-and-coverage-rates-1999-2014-2

Markus, A., Krohe, S., Garro, N., Gerstein, M., & Pellegrini, C. (2017). Examining the association between Medicaid coverage and preterm births using 2010–2013 National Vital Statistics Birth Data. *Journal of Children and Poverty, 23*(1), 79–94. doi:10.1080/10796126.2016.1254601

National Federation of Independent Business v. Sebelius, 567 U.S. 519 (2012). Retrieved from https://www.oyez.org/cases/2011/11-393

New York State. (2015). *Governor Cuomo signs legislation to make New York the first state in the nation to allow pregnant women to enroll in the state health insurance exchange at any time* [Press release]. Retrieved from https://www.governor.ny.gov/news/governor-cuomo-signs-legislation-make-new-york-first-state-nation-allow-pregnant-women-enroll

Organisation for Economic Co-operation and Development. (2014). After decline in U.S. health expenditure growth, OECD sees risk of spending uptick in recovery. Retrieved from http://www.oecd.org/unitedstates/lancet-health-unitedstates.htm

Organisation for Economic Co-operation and Development. (2018). *Members and partners*. Retrieved from http://www.oecd.org/about/membersandpartners

Palanker, D., Volk, J., & Giovannelli, J. (2017). Eliminating essential health benefits will shift financial risk back to consumers. Retrieved from https://www.common wealthfund.org/blog/2017/eliminating-essential-health-benefits-will-shift-financial -risk-back-consumers?redirect_source=/publications/blog/2017/mar/eliminating -essential-health-benefits-financial-risk-consumers

Patient Protection and Affordable Care Act, 42 U.S.C. § 18001 et seq. (2010).

Polsky, D., Cidav, Z., & Swanson, A. (2016). Marketplace plans with narrow physician networks feature lower monthly premiums than plans with larger networks. *Health Affairs, 35*(10), 1842–1848. doi:10.1377/hlthaff.2016.0693

Pregnancy Discrimination Act, 42 U.S.C. § 2000e et seq.

Sawicki, N. (2016). Mandating disclosure of conscience-based limitations on medical practice. *American Journal of Law and Medicine, 42*, 85–128. doi:10.1177/00988588 16644717

Sawyer, B., & Cox, C. (2018). How does health spending in the U.S. compare to other countries? Retrieved from https://www.healthsystemtracker.org/chart-collection/health -spending-u-s-compare-countries/#item-start

Shepherd, K., Platt, E., Franke, K., & Boylan, E. (2017). *Bearing faith: The limits of Catholic health care for women of color*. New York, NY: Columbia Law School. Retrieved from https://www.law.columbia.edu/sites/default/files/microsites/gender-sexuality/ PRPCP/bearingfaith.pdf

Smith, V., Gifford, K., Ellis, E., Edwards, B., Rudowitz, R., Hinton, E., . . . Valentine, A. (2016). *Implementing coverage and payment initiatives: Results from a 50-state Medicaid budget survey for state fiscal years 2016 and 2017*. Retrieved from https:// www.kff.org/medicaid/report/implementing-coverage-and-payment-initiatives -results-from-a-50-state-medicaid-budget-survey-for-state-fiscal-years-2016-and-2017

Sonfield, A. (2016). How and why to integrate reproductive health into delivery system and payment reform. *Guttmacher Policy Review, 19*, 61–66. Retrieved from https:// www.guttmacher.org/gpr/2016/12/how-and-why-integrate-reproductive-health -delivery-system-and-payment-reform

Sonfield, A. (2017). No one benefits if women lose coverage for maternity care. *Guttmacher Policy Review, 20*, 78–81. Retrieved from https://www.guttmacher.org/ gpr/2017/06/no-one-benefits-if-women-lose-coverage-maternity-care

Spurlock, B., & Shannon, M. (2015). The new era of narrow networks: Do they come at the cost of quality? *Health Affairs Blog*. doi:10.1377/hblog20151013.051143

Squires, D. (2015). U.S. health care from a global perspective. Spending, use of services, prices, and health in 13 countries. Retrieved from https://www.commonwealthfund .org/publications/issue-briefs/2015/oct/us-health-care-global-perspective

Stulberg, D., Jackson, R. & Freedman, L. (2016). Referrals for services prohibited in Catholic health care facilities. *Perspectives on Sexual and Reproductive Health, 48*(3), 111–117. doi:10.1363/48e10216

Toland, B. (2014, April 26). How did America end up with this health care system? *Pittsburgh Post-Gazette.* Retrieved from http://www.post-gazette.com/healthypgh/2014/04/27/VITALS-How-did-U-S-employer-based-health-care-history-become-what-it-is-today/stories/201404150167

Turner, W., McKee, C., Chen, A., & Coursolle, A. (2017). *What makes medicaid, medicaid?: Services.* Washington, DC: National Health Law Program. Retrieved from http://www.healthlaw.org/about/staff/wayne-turner/all-publications/what-makes-medicaid-medicaid-services#.WzgbeS2ZMyl

U.S. Conference of Catholic Bishops. (2018). *Ethical and religious directives for Catholic health care services.* Washington, DC: Author. Retrieved from http://www.usccb.org/about/doctrine/ethical-and-religious-directives/upload/ethical-religious-directives-catholic-health-service-sixth-edition-2016-06.pdf

Woolf, S. & Aron, L. (Eds.). (2013). *U.S. health in international perspective: Shorter lives, poorer health.* Washington, DC: National Academies Press.

THE WORKFORCE SHORTAGE AND LIMITED SITES OF CARE

Barriers to Maternal Care

BARBARA A. ANDERSON

OBJECTIVES

At the end of this chapter, the reader will be able to:

1. Describe projections about the shortage of the maternal care workforce and the closure of maternity care sites, especially in rural America.

2. Discuss maternal mortality and severe maternal morbidity in relation to workforce issues and availability of maternity care sites in the United States.

3. Identify current and emerging strategies to develop a diversified workforce and site accessibility for maternal care, especially in rural America.

BARRIERS TO MATERNAL CARE

Shortage of the Maternal Care Workforce in the United States

An effective maternal care workforce is sufficient in numbers, diversified by skills, and appropriately distributed to meet the needs of the population (World Health Organization [WHO], 2015a). The critical issues destabilizing the workforce and creating barriers to maternal care are the increasing need for maternal care providers, both midwives and obstetricians, and the geographical maldistribution of the workforce across the globe (WHO, 2015b). In developed nations, outside of the United States, the average ratio of midwives to obstetricians is 2.5:1 with midwives as the typical provider attending the majority of births and obstetricians managing complications upon referral (Shah, 2015; ten Hoope-Bender et al., 2014). In the United Kingdom, the midwife-to-obstetrician ratio is 19.5:1, and in Australia, it is 16.6:1 (American College of Nurse-Midwives, 2015, as cited in Bradford & Bushman, 2017). In the United States, the ratio of midwives to obstetricians is lower than other developed countries (Association of American Medical Colleges [AAMC], 2014). The workforce shortage in the United States is further exacerbated by declining entrance of medical school graduates into obstetrics/gynecology residencies (Accreditation Council for Graduate Medical Education, 2018; Rayburn, 2017).

In the United States, both shortage and geographical maldistribution of the workforce are increasing, with the greatest impact in Southern and Western regions and rural communities across the nation (Ambrose et al., 2012; Auerbach, Buerhaus, & Staiger, 2017; Clarke, 2016; Ollove, 2016; for further information on the workforce shortage and maldistribution in the United States, see bhw.hrsa.gov/health-workforce-analysis/research).

Categories of the Maternal Care Workforce

The maternal care workforce in the United States includes obstetricians, midwives, family practice physicians, nurse practitioners, physician assistants (PAs), registered nurses working in maternal care, physicians and nurses specialized in anesthesia, and general surgeons performing cesarean section. Doulas are an emerging category of the workforce. In all states, licensed, qualified obstetricians, certified nurse-midwives (CNMs), and family practice doctors can attend births. Not all states allow PAs and certified midwives (CMs) to attend births. There are other categories of midwives, for instance, certified professional midwives (CPMs), who may or may not be prepared, depending upon their background and education, to meet the standards of the International Confederation of Midwives (ICM, 2011; American College of Nurse-Midwives, 2016). These persons may or may not be allowed to provide intrapartal care, depending upon state statutes. With a range of skills that may overlap or be unique to each profession, the cadre of maternal health providers has the potential to offer choice and a collaborative team approach.

Projected Need for Clinicians

The demand for all of these categories of clinicians is projected to increase, with critical needs in states with high population growth, for example, Texas and Florida, in rural areas, and among the growing Hispanic population (Dall, Chakrabarti, Storm, Elwell, & Rayburn, 2013; Rayburn, 2017). The number of births from present to 2060 is estimated to increase by 439,000 (U.S. Census Bureau, 2014).

For the 500,000 rural women giving birth each year, provider shortages are often severe. Currently 40% of all counties in the United States, mostly rural, do not have a provider qualified to attend births (American College of Obstetricians and Gynecologists [ACOG], 2014; Hung, Kozhimannil, Casey, Henning-Smith, & Prasad, 2016; Kozhimannil, Henning-Smith, Hung, Casey, & Prasad, 2016). Without national-level planning for recruitment, retention, retirement, or distribution of the workforce, the vulnerability of populations, including rural mothers, continues (MacLean et al., 2014).

Inadequate Staffing and Closure of Maternity Units

A national trend in the past 20 years has been the closure of maternity care services in rural hospitals. More than 50% of rural hospitals no longer offer obstetrical services (Seigel, 2018). These closures have followed the lack of available maternal care providers and the inability of rural hospitals to ensure adequate staff (Hung, Kozhimannil, Casey, & Moscovice, 2016; Seigel, 2018). Small hospitals with limited workforce are at highest risk for closure of maternity units (Hung, Kozhimannil, Casey, Henning-Smith, & Prasad, 2016; Hung, Kozhimannil, Casey, & Moscovice, 2016).

Increasingly, fewer rural family practice physicians are offering full-scope maternity care services and fewer obstetricians are relocating to rural areas to practice. Many older providers are retiring and replacement is difficult due to isolation, lower salaries, and lack of opportunity for professional advancement. Further, nationwide, many obstetricians do not offer intrapartal services and are subspecializing in gynecology (Jennings, 2015; Kozhimannil et al., 2015; Seigel, 2018). The 500,000 rural births per year in America are spread across a vast geographical area and the volume of births at any one small hospital is low (less than 250 births per year), with fluctuation from year to year (Kozhimannil et al., 2015). Higher volume hospitals, even if rural, are able to attract more obstetricians, midwives, and obstetrical nurses (Kozhimannil et al., 2015).

Scheduling and the need for on-call personnel (obstetricians, midwives, anesthetists, and obstetrical nurses) are difficult with a limited workforce. The institutional burden of maintaining competencies and sufficient expertise is also cited as a reason for maternity unit closures. However, Internet education, mobile high-fidelity simulation units, and telehealth help to bridge the required continuing education gap (Kozhimannil et al., 2015). The most common reason for hospitalization in America is childbirth, but in the current healthcare environment, it is quite expensive for hospitals to offer (Kozhimannil et al., 2016). Nonetheless, the argument can be made that this situation is also an issue of political will. Rural hospitals are able to maintain expensive emergency room services to care for heart attacks and other acute unplanned events. Unpredictable incidents and mass casualty in rural areas have also been well managed by providing rapid services (Bortko, 2019).

The Impact of Workforce Shortage and Limited Sites of Care

Rural women are often at high risk due to poverty, obesity, prepregnancy chronic illnesses, and lack of health insurance. They have four times the risk of adverse outcomes with pregnancy-related complications (Health Resources and Services

Administration [HRSA], 2013; United Nations Human Rights Council [UNHRC], 2018). Limited or no access to maternal care providers or prenatal care and lack of available emergency obstetrical services, increase risk for severe maternal morbidity and double the risk of maternal mortality (ACOG, 2014; Amnesty International, 2011; Bice-Wigington, Simmons, & Huddleston-Casas, 2015; Lazariu, Nguyen, McNutt, Jeffrey, & Kacica, 2017). If care is available, there may be a lack of continuity between locally accessed prenatal care and intrapartal care delivered at a distant site (Hung, Kozhimannil, Casey, Henning-Smith, & Prasad, 2016; Hung, Kozhimannil, Casey, & Moscovice, 2016; Kozhimannil et al., 2015). When staffing is limited, cesarean is more common in rural, low-volume hospitals as a pragmatic solution to safe delivery (Kozhimannil et al., 2014, 2015).

Adverse outcomes are directly proportional to access to maternity care services (Kozhimannil et al., 2015). Over 50% of rural pregnant women live at least 30 minutes to many hours away from a Level 1 hospital offering obstetrical services (Seigel, 2018). Inclement weather conditions, inadequate emergency transport services, and lack of private transportation can further complicate access to care. Of most concern is unattended, unplanned birth in cars, on the roadside, or in local emergency rooms with untrained or minimally obstetrically trained personnel (Hung, Kozhimannil, Casey, Henning-Smith, & Prasad, 2016; Hung, Kozhimannil, Casey, & Moscovice, 2016; Kozhimannil et al., 2015). Emergency transport personnel, while very well trained as first responders, have minimal experience attending births, especially with complications. Neonatal and maternal outcomes can be tragic. There are better solutions as described in the next section.

STRATEGIES TO SUPPORT MATERNAL CARE IN LOW-RESOURCE AREAS

There are both deterrents and incentives for the maternal healthcare workforce to move to rural areas. Multiple strategies have been designed to incentivize and develop a rural workforce, but there are some hard realities to face.

Affordable Liability Insurance

In a remote environment, healthcare providers have latitude, opportunity for innovative practice, and frequently a warm, ongoing relationship with an appreciative community. It is possible to build lifetime friendships and a sense of community. However, it does not always work out that way. Rural health providers face high liability, frequently due to isolation rather than lack of competency. Addressing the inherent risks in rural practice and adjusting for these risks are key elements in encouraging maternal healthcare providers to locate in rural communities.

As an example, low-volume hospitals have higher nonmedically indicated elective primary cesarean section rates and higher elective repeat cesarean delivery (ERCD), sometimes as a pragmatic and defensive stance (Kozhimannil et al., 2014, 2015).

Often, vaginal birth after cesarean (VBAC) section is not offered at rural hospitals due to concern about management of the rare complication of uterine rupture. Repeat cesarean section actually carries greater risk. The evidence from systematic review of VBAC versus ERCD is strong, indicating nine fewer deaths with VBAC than with ERCD (1.9 maternal deaths/100,000 live births with VBAC compared to 9.6/100,000 with ERCD; Guise et al., 2010). The number of maternal deaths is low overall, but it is exacerbated by complicating factors like obesity (Guise et al., 2010), which is common in rural areas (UNHRC, 2018).

In weighing this evidence and considering clinical options, it is important to acknowledge that maternal healthcare providers, often working in isolation and with limited resources, are at high risk for liability. Prevention of primary cesarean section is one important strategy that will be explored in the next chapter. Providing reasonable liability coverage for practitioners in remote areas is another strategy. Oregon passed legislation to provide state income tax credit and assistance with medical liability insurance for rural practitioners. Rural Oregon providers state that these benefits have enabled them to continue providing maternal healthcare in rural areas (ACOG, 2014).

Appropriate Technology to Ensure Competency

Accessing continuing education in rural areas is highly enhanced with technology. Continuing education and online programs are readily accessible for all categories of maternal healthcare providers. Webinars, often featuring interprofessional educational opportunities, as well as locally offered team education can build comradery and a culture of team collaboration. Telehealth offerings are available, not just for patient consultation but also for education. In some places, mobile vans provide high-fidelity simulation learning at a relatively central site. Such educational offerings do more than educate: They create a sense of professional community.

Support for Rural Health Recruitment

Many high- and low-resource nations require students preparing in critical professions to provide at least 1 to 2 years of national service upon completion of their education. This service to the nation, often in remote, high-need areas, can be formative for a young professional. This is not voluntary service; it is required as part of national investment in education. Usually such nations plan for the number of professionals needed based upon population growth, retirement projections, and attrition. Then the government funds part or all of the student's education.

The United States does not have national planning for recruitment, retention, retirement, or distribution of the workforce (MacLean et al., 2014), but there are some incentivizing programs. The U.S. Peace Corps, which is strictly voluntary, collaborates with universities that have various forms of graduate-level internships. I had the immense privilege of serving in the Peace Corps and then bringing formative experiences to lead program development for the U.S. maternal health-care workforce.

The National Health Service Corps

One key program is the National Health Service Corps (NHSC) administered by HRSA through the Bureau of Health Workforce. The NHSC awards scholarships and offers loan repayment programs for workforce development in primary care to designated categories of healthcare providers. There are more than 5,000 communities with provider shortages receiving services from 10,900 primary care providers through the NHSC (HRSA, n.d.).

The NHSC loan repayment program after graduation places qualified primary care, dentistry, and mental health professionals in Health Professional Shortage Areas (HPSAs) after graduation for a 2-year period of service in return for educational loan repayment. The provider can choose the site and HPSAs include rural, urban, tribal, or facility sites (e.g., prisons). A common site is a federally qualified health center (FQHC) providing primary care to underserved population (see HPSAs, https://bhw.hrsa.gov/shortage-designation/hpsas). CNMs, as maternal healthcare providers, are not included in this primary care designation, even though they are board certified to provide primary care of well women (American Midwifery Certification Board, n.d.) This factor is detrimental to providing adequate staffing in isolated areas.

The NHSC scholarship program awards scholarships to students studying to be a physician, a dentist, a nurse practitioner, a CNM, or a PA. This is a full scholarship. The applicant agrees before beginning education to provide 2 years of professional service after graduation in a high-need community (NHSC, n.d.) These government programs, as well as other philanthropic organizations, offer young professionals the opportunity to build knowledge, attitudes, and skills in working with vulnerable, underserved populations, including women in remote and rural areas.

Diversification of the Workforce

One key issue in recruitment is a diversified workforce, not only by skill level and profession (Dawley & Walsh, 2016) but also by ethnic and cultural background, language skills, religious values, and gender identity. Diversification of the workforce begins with serious and sustained efforts to recruit students from multiple ethnicities. It also requires support for scholarships, active recruitment especially at high school and undergraduate level, and sustained support by sensitive faculty, from the ethnic groups represented, as well as from the general pool of faculty. All students need to feel valued and essential to the workforce. In a multicultural nation, America's healthcare workforce needs to reflect the many faces of multiculturalism.

A poignant example of the need for healthcare providers who share cultural values and experiences are those who work with Native Hawaiian and Pacific Islander populations (Ambrose et al., 2012). As an archipelago of islands with logistic challenges, the Hawaiian islands are basically rural. There are narrow, winding roads, often wet from tropical rain, and many miles to the nearest Level 1 healthcare facility. Census tract data and geographical information system (GIS) mapping show maldistribution of the workforce with an urban bias. Providers with crosscutting skills are a strength and a safety net, especially in rural America (Kozhimannil et al., 2015). Even when health providers are available, they are often not from the Native Hawaiian or Pacific Islander population (Ambrose et al., 2012) or from the populations that have settled in the islands for decades. Native Hawaiian cultural values and health practices are often very different from allopathic medical practices (Ambrose et al., 2012).

I have deep family and friendship ties in Hawai'i and have also had the opportunity to be a site visitor for rural facilities providing maternal healthcare: birth centers, home birth sites, and Level 1 hospitals in rural Hawai'i. Like other remote sites, healthcare providers are often isolated, have limited professional opportunities, and receive a relatively low salary. Recruiting and retaining personnel with cultural congruence or who reflect the face of the local population in the beautiful Aloha state is often difficult.

Triage and Risk Assessment for Appropriate Care

An important innovation in maternal healthcare has been the development of the levels-of-care model. This approach places women at an appropriate level of care without neglecting serious conditions or forcing healthy women into unnecessary high-technology settings. It provides a blueprint for regionalization of care with focus on prudent use of resources (Brantley, Davis, Goodman, Callaghan, & Barfield, 2017; Hankins et al., 2012; Menard et al., 2015). The process of triaging mothers for risk has improved but cesarean and denial of low-risk VBAC are often based on lack of access to the appropriate level of care rather than clinical judgment (MacDorman & Declercq, 2016). Menard et al. make the case for an integrated, streamlined, risk-appropriate system with clear expectations of scope of practice at each level (2016). The model, however, does not provide for full utilization of midwifery care at all levels.

This model is built upon the 1976 March of Dimes report, "Toward Improving the Outcome of Pregnancy I," that profoundly improved neonatal care (Rose, 2010). However, the March of Dimes document did not result in focus on maternal levels of care (Hankins et al., 2012). Mothers are often in hospital maternity units that provide care to women with normal birth as well as those with life-threatening pathology. The effect can be a milieu where maternal care providers are necessarily focused on pathology and critically ill women. Normal birth may be secondary to high acuity. The context is often tense, noisy, and unconducive to peaceful family building.

The levels-of-care model addresses appropriate placement of care with attendance by maternal care providers qualified to meet needs. It provides a rubric for critical decision making about the safest and most appropriate settings for physiologic birth, lifesaving care, and maternal conditions and events in between.

All levels of care are responsible for providing appropriate continuing education, competency maintenance, and quality assurance. Each level of care has significant knowledge to contribute in adding to the cumulative knowledge. A positive change in rural areas is the increased utilization of midwifery services (Kozhimannil et al., 2015). A gap in the levels-of-care model is integration of midwifery care at all levels of care. Collaborative midwifery/obstetrician care has been shown to support physiologic birth and to minimize intervention to the extent possible, regardless of level of acuity (Weisband, Klebanoff, Gallo, Shoben, & Norris, 2018; Vedam et al., 2018).

The *Lancet* Series has demonstrated that nations that fully utilize the education and skills of midwives show sustained decrease in maternal mortality (Renfrew et al., 2014). The Institute of Medicine 2010 report, *The Future of Nursing: Leading Change, Advancing Health*, calls on our nation to utilize nursing, the largest cadre of the health professionals in America, to the full scope of education and skills in addressing severe health disparities. Maternal health is part of that disparity. Nurses and midwives have a key role to play in improving maternal health at all levels of care (Committee on the Robert Wood Johnson Foundation Initiative on the Future of Nursing, 2011)

Community-Based Birth

Home Birth

The levels-of-care model as described by Menard et al. (2015) does not include home births. Home birth can be a safe alternative with risk screening, counseling on risk, and appropriate support systems in place. Midwife-attended home birth is part of the National Health Service of many developed nations (Anderson, 2008, 2009; National Institute for Health and Care Excellence [NICE], 2014; Renfrew et al., 2014; Shah, 2015). Planned home birth is a viable solution and the choice of many women, especially in remote areas. I have observed home birth midwifery care and talked with the midwives in the Outback of Australia. The National Health Service supports the process and backstops the midwives with the Flying Doctors, an air ambulance service. This model provides good outcomes and high satisfaction for mothers (Catling-Paull, Coddington, Foureur, & Homer, 2013).

The Birthplace in England National Prospective Cohort Study provides supporting evidence that offering healthy, low-risk women a choice of birth setting, including midwifery-attended home birth, is reasonable (Brocklehurst et al., 2011). All midwives in these high-resource countries are educated to the ICM standards, including American CNMs and CMs (ICM, 2013).

A planned home birth attended by a qualified midwife or family care physician with an appropriately screened low-risk mother can be a lovely birth experience.

It is certainly a better alternative than giving birth in a car or on the roadside. In 2015, there were 36,080 registered home births (Martin, Hamilton, Osterman, Driscoll, & Matthews, 2017). As discussed in the levels-of-care model, a well-designed referral plan with access to emergency transport is essential at each level of acuity. In the United States, frequently there is not a smooth transition plan for access to higher levels of care. Inadequate coordination between providers and sites of care is associated with adverse maternal and newborn outcomes (Vedam et al., 2018). Even when well-designed referral policies for home birth are followed, mothers and their providers are sometimes met with hostility when they access a higher level of care.

The Freestanding Birth Center

The *Lancet* Series (2014), funded by the Gates Foundation, reports that 83% of maternal deaths globally could be averted by scaling up the workforce, in particular midwifery care at the community level (Homer et al., 2014; Kennedy et al., 2018). The workforce pyramid in the United States is inverted toward high-intervention care, expensive and inaccessible to many women, especially in rural America. One solution to cost is freestanding, community-based, midwifery-led birth centers (FSBCs). The Triple Aim, *care, health, and cost*, can be met by providing community-based, high-quality care with proven outcomes (Berwick, Nolan, & Whittington, 2008).

There is a high level of evidence on the efficacy and safety of birth center care in promoting physiologic birth in communities where women live (Alliman & Phillippi, 2016; Alliman, Jolles, & Summers, 2015; Benatar, Garrett, Howell, & Palmer, 2013; Jackson et al., 2003; Rooks et al., 1989; Stapleton, Osborne, & Illuzzi, 2013). Accreditation of FSBCs is well designed and administered by the national accrediting agency, the Commission for the Accreditation of Birth Centers (CABC; n.d.).

Reimbursement for Freestanding Birth Centers

Most private insurances cover birth center facility and provider charges and hospital or physician practices that include birth center/midwifery-led care (American Association of Birth Centers [AABC], 2015). As 50% of all births in the United States are funded by Medicaid, utilization of birth center care would substantially reduce national costs (Alliman et al., 2015; Smith et al., 2017; Torio & Moore, 2016). The Patient Protection and Affordable Care Act (ACA) mandates birth center facility reimbursement and comparable reimbursement for CNMs and physicians through Medicaid (2009). However, Medicaid is administered at the state level and many states have delayed or declined participation in the ACA (Stone, Ernst, & Stapleton, 2017).

One key element of the ACA is coverage for preconceptual screening, primary care, and health education as well as prepregnancy management of conditions that undermine healthy pregnancy (ACA, 2009). In underserved areas, such care is frequently delivered by primary care providers in overextended FQHCs (Xue et al., 2018). This care can be expanded to the FSBC by CNMs and CMs, whose scope of practice includes screening, primary care, and health education of healthy women across the life span (Wilkes & Alliman, 2017). However, in many states, Medicaid reimbursement with ACA-expanded resources to FSBCs continues to be an issue.

Preparing the Workforce

If the reimbursement issue can be resolved, another component of scaling up care in FSBCs is preparing the maternal health workforce to serve in this setting. Most providers are exclusively educated in high-intervention hospital settings and need exposure to this venue during their education (Anderson, Cole, & Bushman, 2017). Knowing how to start and conduct the business of an FSBC is another component. This process is described in detail by Schrag and Anderson (2017). Also, the AABC offers workshops by experienced mentors at multiple sites across the nation. These workshops guide maternal care providers in the steps of starting an FSBC (AABC, n.d.-a).

Example of Birth Center Innovation

In 2012, the Centers for Medicare and Medicaid Services (CMS), the HRSA, and the Administration on Children and Families developed the Strong Start for Mothers and Newborns Initiative with the goal of developing models to improve perinatal outcomes and reduce preterm birth (CMS, 2012). The AABC was awarded a 4-year, $5.5 million grant to evaluate the freestanding-birth-center model in relation to the goals. In 2013, AABC implemented the Strong Start in Birth Centers Initiative in 44 birth centers in 22 states, enhancing care with intensive health education and peer counseling (AABC, n.d.-b). Over the next 4 years, in this particular award, 6,425 women with Medicaid coverage gave birth in these birth centers. CNMs were the most common healthcare providers. The outcomes in these birth centers demonstrated capacity to improve maternal health by decreasing unwarranted intervention, including cesarean, among a diverse, low-risk Medicaid population (Jolles et al., 2017). The 2017 CMS report describes the preliminary outcomes for this national initiative (CMS, 2017).

The final national evaluation, released November 9, 2018, showed a 26% reduction of preterm birth and a cesarean rate of 8.7% with birth center care compared to the national rate of 21.8%. With nulliparous, term, singleton, vertex (NTSV) women, the cesarean rate was 13.9% compared to the national rate of 25.7%. It also demonstrated a $2,010 savings for the 1st year of life for each mother–baby dyad with birth center care, regardless of site of delivery, hospital or birth center (AABC, 2018; CMS, 2017).

Cost reimbursement from Medicaid coverage alone cannot support birth centers. The next step, going forward, is to create a viable cost reimbursement system for birth centers. As of this writing, AABC is proposing national legislation to create a federally funded demonstration project. The Birth Access Benefitting Improved Essential Facility Services (the BABIES Act) would provide birth center care in underserved areas with reimbursement comparable to the federal reimbursement model used by FQHCs. Freestanding birth centers in underserved areas are part of the safety net to increase access to care.

SUMMARY

In the United States, shortage and geographical maldistribution of the maternal care workforce are severe and projected to worsen. The greatest impact is felt in rural communities and in the Southern and Western regions. Increasing access to midwifery care is a critical component in backstopping the maternal care workforce shortage. Other strategies include access for affordable liability insurance, using technology to support care and ensure ongoing competency, educational support for recruitment, and implementing risk assessment/triage for each level of care. As demonstrated in the Strong Start for Mothers and Newborns Initiative, freestanding birth centers can offer a viable solution for a large percentage of rural and underserved low-risk mothers.

WHAT IF

This section poses critical questions and discussion points about the crippling of health and the loss of life among America's mothers. It is an opportunity to think creatively about solutions to the workforce shortage and to the limitations in sites of care. Answers are deliberately not provided. The solutions to this national epidemic lie in interdisciplinary, imaginative conversation and problem solving. The authors invite the readers to consider these questions and add additional ones.

WORKFORCE SHORTAGE AND LIMITED SITES OF CARE: BARRIERS TO MATERNAL CARE

What are some ways to incentivize healthcare providers to choose a maternal health focus?

What are some ways to incentivize healthcare providers to choose rural health practice?

How will webinars, telehealth, Internet continuing education, open-access literature, simulation exercises, and other Internet-based technologies affect healthcare delivery in rural areas?

What social changes would result if the site promoted for normal physiologic birth was the freestanding birth center?

What would the U.S. maternal healthcare system look like if midwives were the preferred provider for normal physiologic birth?

REFERENCES

Accreditation Council for Graduate Medical Education. (2018). *ACGME data resource book 2017–2018.* Available from http://www.acgme.org/acgmeweb/tabid/259/Grad uateMedicalEducation/GraduateMedicalEducationDataResourceBook.aspx

Alliman, J., Jolles, D., & Summers, L. (2015). The innovation imperative: Scaling freestand- ing birth centers, CenteringPregnancy, and midwifery-led maternity health homes. *Journal of Midwifery and Women's Health, 60*(3), 244–249. doi:10.1111/jmwh.12320

Alliman, J., & Phillippi, J. (2016). Maternal outcomes in birth centers: An integrative review of the literature. *Journal of Midwifery and Women's Health, 61*(1), 21–51. doi:10.1111/ jmwh.12356

Ambrose, A., Arakawa, R., Greidanus, B., Macdonald, P., Racsa, P., Shibuya, K., . . . Yamada, S. (2012). Geographical maldistribution of Native Hawaiian and other Pacific Islander Physicians in Hawai'i. *Hawaii Journal of Medicine and Public Health, 71*(4 Suppl. 1), 13–20. Retrieved from https://www.ncbi.nlm.nih.gov/pmc/articles/PMC3347733/pdf/ hjmph7104_suppl1_0013.pdf

American Association of Birth Centers. (n.d.-a). *How to start a birth center: Bringing midwifery to main street.* Retrieved from http://www.birthcenters.org/?page=hsbc _workshops

American Association of Birth Centers. (n.d.-b). Strong Start Initiative for Mothers and New- borns (2013–2017). Retrieved from https://www.birthcenters.org/page/strongstart

American Association of Birth Centers. (2015). Update on AABC Medicaid survey of birth centers. *AABC News.* Retrieved from https://www.birthcenters.org/store/ViewProduct .aspx?ID=10046031

American Association of Birth Centers. (2018, November 9). *New government report recom- mends birth center care* [Press release]. Retrieved from https://www.birthcenters.org/ news/426371/New-Government-Report-Recommends-Birth-Center-Care.htm

American College of Nurse-Midwives. (2016). Legal recognition. Retrieved from http:// www.midwife.org/Legal-Recognition

American College of Obstetricians and Gynecologists Committee on Health Care for Under- served Women. (2014). *Health disparities in rural women* (Committee Opinion No. 586). Retrieved from https://www.acog.org/-/media/Committee-Opinions/Committee-on -Health-Care-for-Underserved-Women/co586.pdf?dmc=1&ts=20160402T0931414521

American Midwifery Certification Board. (n.d.). About American Midwifery Certification Board (AMCB). Retrieved from https://www.amcbmidwife.org/about-amcb

Amnesty International. (2011). *Deadly delivery: The maternal health care crisis in the USA: One-year update.* New York, NY: Amnesty International. Retrieved from https://cdn2 .sph.harvard.edu/wp-content/uploads/sites/32/2017/06/deadlydeliveryoneyear.pdf

Anderson, B. (2008). *Assessment of midwifery practice and birth centers in Denmark, Ice- land, Finland, Norway and Sweden* [Report to the Board of Directors]. Perkiomenville, PA: American Association of Birth Centers. Association of Childbearing Centers.

Anderson, B. (2009, May 2). *Because I have my midwife: A five-country ethnographic study of factors supporting midwifery practice in Scandinavia.* Invited paper presented at American College of Nurse Midwives 54th Annual Convention, Seattle, WA.

Anderson, B., Cole, L., & Bushman, J. (2017). Preparing the workforce. In L. Cole & M. Avery (Eds.), *Freestanding birth centers: Innovation, evidence, optimal outcomes* (pp. 263–284). New York, NY: Springer Publishing Company.

Association of American Medical Colleges. (2014). *2014 physician specialty data book.* Washington, DC: Author. Retrieved from https://www.aamc.org/download/473260/data/2014physicianspecialtydatabook.pdf

Auerbach, D., Buerhaus, P., & Staiger, D. (2017). How fast will the registered nurse workforce grow through 2030? Projections in nine regions of the country. *Nursing Outlook, 65,* 116–122. doi:10.1016/j.outlook.2016.07.004

Benatar, S., Garrett, A., Howell, E., & Palmer, A. (2013). Midwifery care at a freestanding birth center: A safe and effective alternative to conventional maternity care. *Health Services Research, 48*(5), 1750–1768. doi:10.1111/1475-6773.12061

Berwick, D., Nolan, T., & Whittington, J. (2008). The Triple Aim: Care, health, and cost. *Health Affairs, 27*(3), 759–769. doi:10.1377/hlthaff.27.3.759

Bice-Wigington, T., Simmons, L. A., & Huddleston-Casas, C. (2015). An ecological perspective on rural, low-income mothers' health. *Social Work in Public Health, 30*(2), 129–143. doi:10.1080/19371918.2014.969860

Bortko, M. (2019). The effects of gun trauma on rural Montana healthcare providers. In M. deChesnay & B. Anderson (Eds.), *Caring for the vulnerable: Perspectives in nursing theory, practice, and research* (5th ed., pp. 291–301). Burlington, MA: Jones & Bartlett.

Bradford, H., & Bushman, J. (2017). Advocating for childbearing women: Current initiatives and workforce challenges. In B. Anderson, J. Rooks, & R. Barroso (Eds.), *Best practices in midwifery: Using the evidence to implement change* (2nd ed., pp. 23–49). New York, NY: Springer Publishing Company.

Brantley, M., Davis, N., Goodman, D., Callaghan, W., & Barfield, W. (2017). Perinatal regionalization: A geospatial view of perinatal critical care, United States, 2010–2013. *American Journal of Obstetrics and Gynecology, 216*(185), 185.e1–185.e10. doi:10.1016/j.ajog.2016.10.011

Brocklehurst, P., Hardy, P., Hollowell, J., Linsell, L., Macfarlane, A., McCourt, C., . . . Stewart, M. (2011). Perinatal and maternal outcomes by planned place of birth for healthy women with low risk pregnancies: The Birthplace in England national retrospective cohort study. *British Medical Journal, 343,* d7400. doi:10.1136/bmj.d7400

Catling-Paull, C., Coddington, R. L., Foureur, M. J., & Homer, C. S. (2013). Publicly funded homebirth in Australia: A review of maternal and neonatal outcomes over 6 years. *Medical Journal of Australia, 198*(11), 616–620. doi:10.5694/mja12.11665

Centers for Medicare and Medicaid Services. (2012, July 3). *Strong start for mothers and newborns: Fact sheet.* Retrieved from https://innovation.cms.gov/initiatives/strong-start/strong-start-for-mothers-and-newborns-fact-sheet.html

Centers for Medicare and Medicaid Services. (2017). *Strong start for mothers and newborns initiative: General information.* Center for Medicare and Medicaid Innovation. Retrieved from https://innovation.cms.gov/initiatives/strong-start

Clarke, S. (2016). RN workforce update: Current and long-range forecast. *Nursing Management, 47*(11), 20–25. doi:10.1097/01.NUMA.0000502798.99305.10

Commission for the Accreditation of Birth Centers. (n.d.). *Accredited birth centers.* Retrieved from https://www.birthcenteraccreditation.org/find-accredited-birth-centers

Committee on the Robert Wood Johnson Foundation Initiative on the Future of Nursing. (2011). *The future of nursing: Leading change, advancing health.* Washington, DC: National Academies Press.

Dall, T., Chakrabarti, R., Storm, M., Elwell, E., & Rayburn, W. (2013). Estimated demand for women's health services by 2020. *Journal of Women's Health, 22*(7), 643–648. doi:10.1089/jwh.2012.4119

Dawley, K., & Walsh, L. (2016). Creating a more diverse midwifery workforce in the United States: A historical reflection. *Journal of Midwifery and Women's Health, 61*(5), 578–585. doi:10.1111/jmwh.12489

Guise, J.-M., Eden, K., Emeis, C., Denman, M. A., Marshall, N., Fu, R., . . . McDonagh, M. (2010). *Vaginal birth after cesarean: New insights* (Evidence Report/Technology Assessment No. 191, AHRQ Publication No. 10-E003). Rockville, MD: Agency for Healthcare Research and Quality.

Hankins, G., Clark, S., Pacheco, L., O'Keeffe, D., D'Alton, M., & Saade, G. (2012). Maternal mortality, near misses, and severe morbidity: Lowering rates through designated levels of maternity care. *Obstetrics and Gynecology, 120*(4), 929–934. doi:10.1097/AOG.0b013e31826af878

Health Resources and Services Administration. (2013). *Child health USA 2013.* Rockville, MD: U.S. Department of Health and Human Services. Retrieved from https://mchb.hrsa.gov/chusa13/dl/pdf/chusa13.pdf

Hill, I., Benatar, S., Courtot, B., Dubay, L., Blavin, F., Garrett, B., . . . Sinnarajah, B. (2017). *Strong Start for Mothers and Newborns evaluation: Year 3 annual report.* Washington, DC: Urban Institute.

Homer, C., Friberg, I., Bastos Dias, M., ten Hoope-Bender, P., Sandall, J., Speciale, A., & Bartlett, L. (2014). The projected effect of scaling up midwifery. *Lancet, 384*(9948), 1146–1157. doi:10.1016/S0140-6736(14)60790-X

Hung, P., Kozhimannil, K., Casey, M., Henning-Smith, C., & Prasad, S. (2016). *State variations in the rural obstetric workforce.* Minneapolis: University of Minnesota Rural Health Research Center. Retrieved from http://rhrc.umn.edu/wp-content/uploads/2016/05/State-Variations-in-the-Rural-Obstetric-Workforce.pdf

Hung, P., Kozhimannil, K., Casey, M., & Moscovice, I. (2016). Why are obstetric units in rural hospitals closing their doors? *Health Services Research, 51*(4), 1546–1560. doi:10.1111/1475-6773.12441

International Confederation of Midwives. (2011). *Definition of the midwife.* Retrieved from https://www.internationalmidwives.org/our-work/policy-and-practice/icm-defini tions.html

International Confederation of Midwives. (2013). *Global standards for midwifery education, with companion guidelines* (ICM Core Document 2010, amended 2013). Retrieved from https://www.internationalmidwives.org/assets/files/general-files/2018/04/com panion-guidelines-for-ed-standards-2011---amended-web-edition-june-2013.pdf

Jackson, D., Lang, J., Swartz, W., Ganiats, T., Fullerton, J., Ecker, J., & Nguyen, U. (2003). Outcomes, safety, and resource utilization in a collaborative care birth center program compared with traditional physician-based perinatal care. *American Journal of Public Health, 93*(6), 999–1006. doi:10.2105/AJPH.93.6.999

Jennings, J. C. (2015). Women's healthcare: Initiatives and challenges. *Women's Health, 11*(6), 801–804. doi:10.2217/whe.15.36

Jolles, D., Langford, R., Stapleton, S., Cesario, S., Koci, A., & Alliman, J. (2017). Outcomes of childbearing Medicaid beneficiaries engaged in care at Strong Start birth center sites between 2012 and 2014. *Birth, 44*(4), 298–305. doi:10.1111/birt.12302

Kennedy, H., Cheyney, M., Dahlen, H., Downe, S., Foureur, M., Homer, C., . . . Renfrew, M. (2018). Asking different questions: A call to action for research to improve the quality of care for every woman, every child. *Birth, 45*(3), 222–231. doi:10.1111/birt .12361

Kozhimannil, K., Casey, M., Hung, P., Han, X., Prasad, S., & Moscovice, I. (2015). The rural obstetric workforce in US Hospitals: Challenges and opportunities. *Journal of Rural Health, 31*(4), 365–372. doi:10.1111/jrh.12112

Kozhimannil, K., Henning-Smith, C., Hung, P., Casey, M., & Prasad, S. (2016). Ensuring access to high-quality maternity care in rural America. *Women's Health Issues, 26*(3), 247–250. doi:10.1016/j.whi.2016.02.001

Kozhimannil, K., Hung, P., Prasad, S., Casey, M., McClellan, M., & Moscovice, I. (2014). Birth volume and the quality of obstetric care in rural hospitals. *Journal of Rural Health, 30*(4), 335–343. doi:10.1111/jrh.12061

Lazariu, V., Nguyen, T., McNutt, L.-A., Jeffrey, J., & Kacica, M. (2017). Severe maternal morbidity: A population-based study of an expanded measure and associated factors. *PLoS ONE, 12*(8), e0182343. doi:10.1371/journal.pone.0182343

MacDorman, M., & Declercq, E. (2016). Trends and characteristics of United States out-of-hospital births 2004–2014: New information on risk status and access to care. *Birth, 43*(2), 116–124. doi:10.1111/birt.12228

MacLean, L., Hassmiller, S., Shaffer, F., Rohrbaugh, K., Collier, T., & Fairman, J. (2014). Scale, causes, and implications of the primary care nursing shortage. *Annual Review of Public Health, 35*, 443–457. doi:10.1146/annurev publhealth 032013 182508

Martin, J., Hamilton, B., Osterman, M., Driscoll, A., & Matthews, T. (2017). Births: Final data for 2015. *National Vital Statistics Reports, 66*(1), 1–69. Retrieved from https:// www.cdc.gov/nchs/data/nvsr/nvsr66/nvsr66_01.pdf

Menard, K., Kilpatrick, S., Saade, G., Hollier, L., Joseph, G., Jr., Barfield, W., . . . Conry, J. (2015). Levels of maternal care. *American Journal of Obstetrics and Gynecology, 212*(3), 259–271. doi:10.1016/j.ajog.2014.12.030

National Health Service Corps. (n.d.). How to comply with scholarship program requirements. Retrieved from https://nhsc.hrsa.gov/scholarships/requirements-compliance.html

National Institute for Health and Care Excellence. (2014). *Intrapartum care for healthy women and their babies.* Retrieved from http://www.nice.org.uk/guidance/cg190/chapter/1 -recommendations

Ollove, M. (2016). *A shortage in the nation's maternal health care.* Retrieved from http://www.pewtrusts.org/en/research-and-analysis/blogs/stateline/2016/08/15/a-shortage -in-the-nations-maternal-health-care

Patient Protection and Affordable Care Act, 42 U.S.C. § 18001 et seq. (2010).

Rayburn, W. (2017). *The obstetrician–gynecologist workforce in the US: Facts, figures, and implications.* Washington, DC: American Congress of Obstetricians and Gynecologists.

Renfrew, M. J., McFadden, A., Bastos, M. H., Campbell, J., Channon, A. A., Cheung, N. F., . . . Declercq, E. (2014). Midwifery and quality care: Findings from a new evidence-informed framework for maternal and newborn care. *Lancet, 384*(9948), 1129–1145. doi:10.1016/S0140-6736(14)60789-3

Rooks, J. P., Weatherby, N. L., Ernst, E. K., Stapleton, S., Rosen, D., & Rosenfield, A. (1989). Outcomes of care in birth centers: National birth center study. *New England Journal of Medicine, 321*(26), 1804–1811. doi:10.1056/NEJM198912283212606

Rose, D., (2010). A history of the March of Dimes. Retrieved from https://www.marchof dimes.org/mission/a-history-of-the-march-of-dimes.aspx

Schrag, K., & Anderson, B. (2017). Creating a birth center: Entrepreneurial midwifery. In B. Anderson, J. Rooks, & R. Barroso (Eds.), *Best practices in midwifery: Using the evidence to implement change* (2nd ed., pp. 283–298). New York, NY: Springer Publishing Company.

Seigel, J. (2018, March 7). Delivering rural babies: Maternity care shortages in rural America. *Rural Health Voices.* Retrieved from https://www.ruralhealthweb.org/blogs/ruralhealthvoices/march-2018/delivering-rural-babies-maternity-care-shortages

Shah, N. (2015). A NICE delivery—The cross-Atlantic divide over treatment intensity in childbirth. *New England Journal of Medicine, 372*(23), 2181–2183. doi:10.1056/NEJMp1501461

Smith, V., Gifford, K., Ellis, E., Edwards, B., Rudowitz, R., Hinton, E., . . . Valentine, A. (2017). *Implementing coverage and payment initiatives: Results from a 50-state Medicaid budget survey for state fiscal years 2016 and 2017.* Retrieved from https://www.kff.org/medicaid/report/implementing-coverage-and-payment-initiatives-results -from-a-50-state-medicaid-budget-survey-for-state-fiscal-years-2016-and-2017

Stapleton, S., Osborne, C., & Illuzzi, J. (2013). Outcomes of care in birth centers: Demonstration of a durable model. *Journal of Midwifery and Women's Health, 58*(1), 3–14. doi:10.1111/jmwh.12003

Stone, S., Ernst, E., & Stapleton, S. (2017). The freestanding birth center: Evidence for change in the delivery of health care to childbearing families. In B. Anderson, J. Rooks, & R. Barroso (Eds.), *Best practices in midwifery: Using the evidence to implement change* (2nd ed., pp. 261–282). New York, NY: Springer Publishing Company.

ten Hoope-Bender, P., de Bernis, L., Campbell, J., Downe, S., Fauveau, V., Fogstad, H., . . . Van Lerberghe, W. (2014). Improvement of maternal and newborn health through midwifery. *Lancet, 384*(9949), 1226–1235. doi:10.1016/S0140-6736(14)60930-2

Torio, C., & Moore, B. (2016). *National inpatient hospital costs: The most expensive conditions by payer, 2013.* Retrieved from https://www.hcup-us.ahrq.gov/reports/statbriefs/sb204-Most-Expensive-Hospital-Conditions.jsp

United Nations Human Rights Council. (2018). *Report of the Special Rapporteur on extreme poverty and human rights on his mission to the United States of America.* Retrieved from https://digitallibrary.un.org/record/1629536/files/A_HRC_38_33_Add-1-EN.pdf

United States Census Bureau. (2014). *2014 National Population Projections.* Retrieved from https://www.census.gov/data/datasets/2014/demo/popproj/2014-popproj.html

Vedam, S., Stoll, K., MacDorman, M., Declercq, E., Cramer, R., Cheyney, M., . . . Kennedy, H. (2018). Mapping integration of midwives across the United States: Impact on access, equity, and outcomes. *PLoS ONE, 13*(2), e0192523. doi:10.1371/journal.pone.0192523

Weisband, Y., Klebanoff, M., Gallo, M., Shoben, A., & Norris, A. (2018). Birth outcomes of women using a midwife versus women using a physician for prenatal care. *Journal of Midwifery and Women's Health, 63*(4), 399–409. doi:10.1111/jmwh.12750

Wilkes, A., & Alliman, J. (2017). Enhanced care services and health homes. In L. Cole & M. Avery (Eds.), *Freestanding birth centers: Innovation, evidence, optimal outcomes* (pp. 229–247). New York, NY: Springer Publishing Company.

World Health Organization. (2015a). *Health workforce 2030: Towards a global strategy on human resources for health.* Geneva, Switzerland: Author. Retrieved from http://www.who.int/hrh/documents/15-295Strategy_Report-04_24_2015.pdf?ua=1

World Health Organization. (2015b). *World health statistics 2015: Part II: Global health indicators.* Geneva, Switzerland: Author. Retrieved from http://www.who.int/gho/publications/world_health_statistics/EN_WHS2015_Part2.pdf?ua=1

Xue, Y., Greener, E., Kannan, V., Smith, J., Brewer, C., & Spetz, J. (2018). Federally qualified health centers reduce the primary care provider gap in health professional shortage counties. *Nursing Outlook, 66*(3), 263–272. doi:10.1016/j.outlook.2018.02.003

EQUITY IN CLINICAL CARE

Addressing the Social Determinants of Maternal Health

BARBARA A. ANDERSON | JENNIFER FOSTER

OBJECTIVES

At the end of this chapter, the reader will be able to:

1. Identify how maternal health in the United States can be enhanced by providing an environment of social justice and equity.

2. Discuss priority areas of clinical care essential to addressing the social determinants of the maternal health crisis in the United States.

3. Describe selected evidence-based initiatives to promote equity and standardization of care in the prevention of maternal mortality and the management of severe maternal morbidity in the United States.

CHANGING THE PARADIGM IN CLINICAL CARE

The United States has poorer health and decreased longevity compared to other nations in the world (Woolf & Aron, 2013). American mothers are no exception to this national profile. *Healthy People* is the 10-year national agenda that identifies major threats to health and longevity among the American population. With broad input from organizations across the nation, this blueprint for action is a comprehensive plan of risk reduction and health promotion (Division for Heart Disease and Stroke Prevention, n.d.). The overarching goal is attainment of health equity for the American population with special attention to the social determinants that create health disparity (Office of Disease Prevention and Health Promotion, n.d.).

Healthy People 2020 addresses the maternal health crisis. National priorities are reduction of maternal mortality, decline in the number of cesarean births among low-risk mothers, and decrease in severe maternal morbidity (National

Conference of State Legislatures, 2011). Mothers at highest risk for mortality and severe morbidity are often those women with many undermining social determinants of health, for example, poverty, lack of access to healthcare, geographical isolation, cultural and racial discrimination, mental health issues, and exposure to violence. Up to 60% of maternal mortality could be prevented by modifying these social factors at the base of the Health Impact Pyramid (Braveman & Gottlieb, 2014; Building U.S. Capacity to Review and Prevent Maternal Deaths, 2018; Centers for Disease Control and Prevention [CDC], 2013).

The traditional pattern of clinical care for antenatal, intrapartal, and postpartum care is based upon templates of practice that frequently do not consider the disruption and danger of undermining social determinants. One example of severe disparity and inequity is hunger (Gany et al., 2014). Among pregnant women, food security is critical to health and may be an immediate problem, not when Medicaid for Pregnancy, the special funding for uninsured pregnant women, becomes available. Thinking from the paradigm of social determinants, rather than templates of practice, hunger needs to be addressed as a priority, cutting through bureaucratic paperwork at Medicaid intake and taking precedent over routine care.

Policy makers, social scientists, public health educators, and health providers agree that health equity can be achieved only if deliberative actions to disrupt undermining social determinants are the focus of care, not an afterthought (Association for Prevention Teaching and Research [APTR], 2018; Byhoff et al., 2017; Hughes, 2016; Kozhimannil, Vogelsang, Hardeman, & Prasad, 2016; Institute of Medicine [IOM], 2011). Such actions require coordinated policy, full scope of practice among health professionals, especially nurses, and interdisciplinary education of both practitioners and students from multiple disciplines (APTR, 2018; Interprofessional Education Collaborative Expert Panel, 2011; IOM, 2011; Reeves, Perrier, Goldman, Feeth, & Zwarenstein, 2013).

In this chapter, the focus is on addressing clinical care from the framework of social determinants, proposing strategies grounded in the literature of healthcare, public health, and the social sciences. Disrupting undermining social determinants needs to be the paradigm of care. This paradigm is presented from four vantage points:

- Embracing equity
- Safeguarding respectful birth and physiologic care
- Reducing cesarean birth
- Preventing and managing risk

EMBRACING EQUITY

Philosopher John Rawls, looking to the work of Immanuel Kant, developed the theory of "justice as fairness," defining the well-ordered society as characterized by the just distribution of goods, with special attention to the most vulnerable

(Rawls, 1971). Building upon justice as fairness, the concept of "health justice" emerged. It is defined as equitable availability and provision of healthcare, a safety net backed up by judicial and legislative bodies responsible for protecting the health of the public (Benfer, 2015). When mothers die or suffer because they are exposed to discrimination, racism, or implicit bias, the safety net is torn. Reducing maternal mortality and morbidity requires all parties involved in healthcare to exert political will for healthcare equity.

Healthcare Equity

Structural violence, cultural/racial discrimination, and implicit bias are the pervasive lived experience of many American mothers. The most vulnerable mothers in America are those who experience the greatest impact of American cultural and historical racism. Healthcare systems and providers are in key positions to embrace and model a culture of justice and health equity. Unfortunately, sometimes they are the problem, demonstrating implicit bias and basing healthcare decisions on stereotypes and assumptions about race (Williams, 2016).

The *Proceedings of the National Academy of Sciences* recently published a disturbing analysis showing that lay Whites as well as 50% of White medical students and medical residents held incorrect biological assumptions of diminished pain sensations among African Americans compared to Whites. Those health providers holding incorrect assumptions about pain consistently made inaccurate and fewer recommendations for pain management among African American patients. However, those free of this belief showed no bias in treatment of pain between African Americans and Whites. This finding is an excellent example of the impact of discrimination and implicit bias on a vulnerable population (Hoffman, Trawalter, Axt, & Oliver, 2016).

There is ample literature addressing the inadequate uptake and continuity of prenatal care among mothers who have poor relationships with their healthcare providers (D'Angelo, Bryan, & Kurz, 2015). Among African American and Hispanic women, 20% report discriminatory treatment by staff during hospitalization for birth (Childbirth Connection, 2018). Conversely, uninterrupted care is most likely among mothers who trust and are satisfied with their healthcare providers, especially among those mothers most at risk for racism (Edmonds, Mogul, & Shea, 2015; Gadson, Akpovi, & Mehta, 2017; Mazul, Salm Ward, & Ngui, 2017).

Creating a Healthcare Culture of Equity

Implicit bias, even the subtlest cues of nonverbal communication, can send powerful discriminatory messages. Many verbal expressions in everyday language are not consciously considered or even meant to be hostile. They are simply cultural manifestation of the pervasive effect of historical racism and White privilege in America. An example of explicit bias is the term "diverse populations" when used as a code for minorities. Defining a group as "diverse" benchmarks that group against "normative." Creating an equitable healthcare environment requires changing the way we look at each other and the way we talk with and about each other. Some resources to understanding the dynamics of racism, privilege, power, and inequity are identified in Table 6.1.

TABLE 6.1 Dynamics of Racism, Privilege, Power, and Inequity: Resources

TITLE	SOURCE	DESCRIPTION
DiAngelo, R. (2011) White fragility	*International Journal of Critical Pedagogy, 3*(3), 54–70	Examines the insulation and comfort zone of Whites that inhibits the ability to tolerate racial stress and creates a sense of fragility
Fine, A., & Kotelchuck, M. (2010) *Rethinking MCH: The life course model as an organizing work*	Department of Health and Human Services, Rockville, MD. Retrieved from https://www.hrsa.gov/sites/default/files/ourstories/mchb75th/images/rethinkingmch.pdf	Examines life course theory as a basis for identifying social determinants
Harvard University (2011) *Project Implicit*	https://implicit.harvard.edu/implicit/education.html	Implicit association test (IAT) measures attitudes and beliefs about bias
Howell, E., & Gobman, W. (2016) *Reduction in peripartum racial/ethnic disparities: Patient safety bundle*	Counsel of Patient Safety in Women's Health, Safety Action Series. Retrieved from www.safehealthcareforeverywoman.org	PowerPoint on impact of racial/ethnic disparities on the health of childbearing women
Roberts, D. (2015) *The problem with race-based medicine*	TED Talk, Palm Springs, CA. Retrieved from https://www.ted.com/talks/dorothy_roberts_the_problem_with_race_based_medicine	Describes how race is an attributed factor in diagnosis and treatment
Sue, W. (2015) *Race talk and the conspiracy of silence: Understanding and facilitating difficult dialogues on race*	Hoboken, NJ: John Wiley & Sons	Examines race talk and offers ways to have the conversation
Teaching Tolerance Test yourself for hidden bias	Retrieved from https://www.tolerance.org/professional-development/test-yourself-for-hidden-bias	Discusses implicit bias and ways to identify it
Williams, D. (2016) *How racism makes us sick*	TED Talk. Retrieved from https://www.ted.com/talks/david_r_williams_how_racism_makes_us_sick	Presents the allostatic stress effects of racism on a person's health over time

A recent article in the *New England Journal of Medicine* discussed learning strategies to help health professionals promote health equity. Some of the learning constructs include:

- Understanding the semantic difference between "race" as a social construct and "racism" as a system that creates inequity

- Learning about the often-untold history of racism in America

- Recognizing and calling out racism

- Practicing self-awareness about historical and contemporary factors influencing clinical care and defining "normal" (Hardeman, Medina, & Kozhimannil, 2016)

As of this writing, the Senate bill, Maternal Care Access and Reducing Emergencies (CARE) Act, introduced by Senator Kamala Harris (California), calls for $30 million in annual grants to train healthcare professionals in recognizing and attending to the issues of implicit bias, racism, and racial disparity in maternal health outcomes (Haberkorn, 2018). In the current political climate, the bill raises awareness but may not have a strong chance of success. Another endeavor is the work of the APTR (see www.teachpopulationhealth.org). APTR developed the Clinical Prevention and Population Health Curriculum Framework, a core curriculum designed as an educational tool for health professional students and practicing health professionals. The case studies in this multiuniversity interprofessional curriculum are very interactive. One case study applicable to this chapter is Seeking Health Equity: Examining Racism as a Social Determinant of Health, and it uses actual situations that demonstrate the impact of racism on health (Yongue, Caiola, & Dixon, 2017).

A strategy in building a culture of health equity is the use of "safety bundles," systematic protocols to direct care and create system-level change. One of the important bundles addresses building health equity through reduction in racial and ethnic disparities (American College of Obstetricians and Gynecologists [ACOG], 2016b). Creating health equity is a cultural journey that requires collective and individual reflection. Anyone, regardless of self-identified race or ethnicity, can hold incorrect assumptions about the *other*. Awareness and moving away from one's biases are journeys of courage that all health professionals need to take.

Creating Equity Through a Culture of Safety

One way of creating equity for mothers is through promoting a culture of safety. In 2006, the California Maternal Quality Care Collaborative (CMQCC) was founded in response to rising maternal mortality and morbidity in the state. In collaboration with the March of Dimes and the California Department of Health, CMQCC quickly responded by developing toolkits with consistent management approaches for providers, guidance to hospitals in quality improvement approaches, and consumer education (CMQCC, n.d.-a). California's maternal mortality declined

by 55% within 7 years (CMQCC, n.d.-b). At present, California has the best maternal mortality statistics in the nation (4.5/100,000 live births), matching developed
nations and meeting World Health Organization (WHO) goals (Agrawal, 2015;
CDC, 2018).

Nonetheless, maternal mortality has escalated around the nation. Amnesty International (2011) shocked the nation with documentation related to inconsistent
management of obstetrical emergencies, lack of coordination of care, increasing
comorbidity during childbearing, and inadequate data retrieval and management.
The concept of protocol-driven maternal safety bundles spread across the nation as
states looked to the California model.

Maternal Safety Bundles and Tools

Coalitions developed as evidence-based management protocols were developed.
The Council on Patient Safety in Women's Health Care is a consortium of organizations involved with the health of women. It publishes web-based tools, including interactive teleconferences, toolkits for evaluating events, and a standardized
template for safety bundles (Box 6.1). The Safety Action Series provides interactive teleconference offerings and the Patient Safety Tools offer guidance on how to
evaluate events. Standardized safety bundles provide an organized structure with
common terminology. This open-access material is based upon established best
practices. Each maternal safety bundle includes:

- A downloadable PDF of the bundle
- A listing of resources
- Live webcast presentation with saved audio and PowerPoint material
- Link to current professional publications describing use of each specific
  bundle
- The designated bundle on the individual home page
- A listing of all current and available maternal safety bundles

Each maternal safety bundle comprises four sections. The *Readiness* section includes information that a healthcare system needs to convey to patients and families. It suggests how to organize a health service to meet this need and lists resources.
Next is the *Recognition and Prevention* section, which identifies specific resources
to prevent and recognize an adverse maternal health problem. The *Response* section
addresses the key elements and resources needed to manage such an event. Lastly,
the *Reporting/Systems Learning* section offers guidelines for developing a reporting
system and disseminating learning.

Alliance for Innovation on Maternal Health

This initiative, AIM, seeks to improve maternal safety and reduce maternal mortality. It has developed national-level networks and education on timely, accessible

---

BOX 6.1

MATERNAL SAFETY BUNDLES AND PATIENT SAFETY TOOLS

MATERNAL SAFETY BUNDLES

The designation +AIM on a maternal safety bundle indicates collaboration and approval by AIM.

- Maternal Mental Health: Depression and Anxiety
- Maternal Venous Thromboembolism (+AIM)
- Obstetric Care for Women With Opioid Use Disorder (+AIM)
- Obstetric Hemorrhage (+AIM)
- Postpartum Care Basics for Maternal Safety: Transition From Maternity to Well-Woman Care (+AIM)
- Postpartum Care Basics for Maternal Safety: From Birth to the Comprehensive Postpartum Visit (+AIM)
- Prevention of Retained Vaginal Sponges After Birth
- Reduction of Peripartum Racial/Ethnic Disparities (+AIM)
- Safe Reduction of Primary Cesarean Birth (+AIM)
- Severe Hypertension in Pregnancy (+AIM)
- Support After a Severe Maternal Event (+AIM)

PATIENT SAFETY TOOLS

- Maternal Early Warning Criteria
  Maternal Early Warning Signs Protocol PDF
- Severe Maternal Morbidity Forms
  Severe Maternal Morbidity Review (+AIM)
  Summary After a Severe Maternal Event (+AIM)

AIM, Alliance for Innovation on Maternal Health.

SOURCE: The Council on Patient Safety in Women's Health Care. (n.d.). Patient safety bundles. Retrieved from https://safehealthcareforeverywoman.org/patient-safety-bundles

---

responses from the healthcare system (AIM, 2015). AIM works with the Council on Patient Safety in Women's Health and provides expert guidance based upon evidence-based best practices. In addition to American College of Obstetricians and Gynecologists (ACOG), the AIM core partnership group includes:

- American College of Nurse-Midwives (ACNM)
- ACOG

- Association of Maternal and Child Health Programs (AMCHP)

- Association of State and Territorial Health Officials (ASTHO)

- Association of Women's Health, Obstetric, and Neonatal Nurses (AWHONN)

- CMQCC

- Society for Maternal–Fetal Medicine (SMFM)

- The Health Resources and Services Administration Maternal and Child Health Bureau (HRSA-MCHB; AIM, 2015)

Support for Creating a Culture of Safety

The Institute for Healthcare Improvement, with support from the $500 million Merck for Mothers program, has initiated a 3-year program to address maternal morbidity and mortality. Promoting the maternal safety bundles and toolkits is a primary strategy in creating a culture of equity and safety (Institute for Healthcare Improvement, n.d.). However, only about 40% of hospitals have adopted the +AIM maternal safety bundles (CBS News, 2018). The challenge is convincing hospitals and providers to accept and implement the bundles.

Condition-specific protocols, in general, do not necessarily improve outcomes. In a 3-year cohort study of 25 hospitals examining a wide range of protocols and implementation strategies on hemorrhage, shoulder dystocia, and preeclampsia, the only condition improved by protocol was preeclampsia. The investigators acknowledge that the quality of these protocols was not assessed, nor was the impact of varying levels of implementation. The study concludes that protocols make no difference and should not be a regulatory factor in practice. The study also concludes that further research is needed to identify the elements of a high-quality protocol and the best implementation strategies (Bailit et al., 2016).

Research is needed to evaluate the effectiveness of toolkits and safety bundles, controlling for protocol design and implementation strategies. The CMQCC toolkits and +AIM safety bundles have been carefully designed by leading experts in maternal health. Institutional support for implementation of high-quality protocols may be a determining factor with respect to outcomes. A good example is the work of an academic medical center team in Brooklyn, New York. A protocol on creating a "culture of mutual respect" was successfully implemented in the operating rooms. The authors note the challenges of entrenched behaviors, the need for institutional leadership and support, and a realistic plan to allow time for change (Kaplan, Mestel, & Feldman, 2010).

A culture of safety is an environment that is built upon equity and respectful care. Healthcare systems and providers have a responsibility to foster this kind of inclusive, just environment. Each mother brings her unique life story to childbearing as explained by life course theory. Much of her story is grounded in the social determinants of health and may include adverse life experiences. It is not uncommon for a pregnant woman to have experiences of poverty, racism, childhood abuse, mental illness, illicit drug use, depression, and intimate partner violence. These adverse life experiences are part of the fabric of her story, often taking a toll on her health. In the face of these adversities, respectful care may be a critical determinant as to how she births, whether she thrives, or if she survives.

SAFEGUARDING RESPECTFUL BIRTH AND PHYSIOLOGIC CARE

Creating equity helps to ensure that every woman is cared for respectfully during her childbearing experience, empowering her inherent ability to create new life. ACNM has developed the Healthy Birth Initiative, promoting physiologic birth (see www.midwife.org/ACNM-Healthy-Birth-Initiative). The midwifery consensus statement by ACNM, the Midwives Alliance of North America (MANA), and the National Association of Certified Professional Midwives (NACPM) identifies key interventions that have been shown to interrupt the physiologic process of birth. These include, but are not limited to, nutritional deprivation of food and fluids and induction or augmentation of labor with synthetic oxytocin (ACNM, MANA, & NACPM, 2012). Both ACNM and ACOG have issued position statements in support of physiologic birth (ACNM, MANA, & NACPM, 2012; ACOG, 2017a).

Promoting Physiologic Labor and Birth

Physiologic childbearing is the innate capacity of the woman to give birth to her child. Women, especially those with low health literacy, may not understand the concept of physiologic birth or believe in their own capacity to achieve it. This understanding requires preparation antenatally, with ample communication between women and the healthcare staff about the primary value of physiologic birth in reducing risk and enhancing health. Environments and interventions that disrupt the physiological process may produce a cascade of complications for either the mother or her newborn or both (Sakara, Romano, & Buckley, 2016). A key message for women is that the routine use of high-technology interventions for every birthing mother is not beneficial, while acknowledging the benefits in complicated births (King & Pinger, 2014). Moreover, women need to be informed that achievement of physiologic birth is not an all-or-nothing phenomenon. While some women may have a solid medical indication for interventions, excellence in clinical care can support their capacities for participating in the birth to the fullest extent possible.

Frequent comorbidities among American mothers have driven routine triage of low- and high-risk women, sometimes as exclusive categories. Once assigned to a high-risk status, physiologic birth and any level of participation may be sidelined, despite the evidence of benefit. A high-risk woman may lose confidence in her capacity to participate at any level in giving birth. Providers may convey this message implicitly or explicitly. Given that more than 98% of women in the United States give birth in hospitals (MacDorman & Declercq, 2016), a hospital environment supportive of physiologic birth and participation to the fullest extent is important for all pregnant women, whether or not they are high risk.

Induction of labor can interfere with the physiologic process. The administration of synthetic oxytocin may desensitize the receptors of endogenous oxytocin, which can slow the progress of the first- or second-stage labor. Prolonged exposure to exogenous oxytocin may increase risk for postpartum hemorrhage, since the endogenous receptors for uterine contraction may not function normally in the presence of exogeneous synthetic oxytocin (Sakara et al., 2016). In the United States, 41% of women have labor induced with synthetic oxytocin (Declercq, Sakala, Corry, Applebaum, & Herrlich, 2013).

Of particular concern is elective (without medical or obstetrical rationale) early induction prior to 39 weeks' gestation. Early induction is associated with increased neonatal morbidities without benefit to the mother (Main et al., 2010). The rate of elective induction has increased in the last decade. The CMQCC has a toolkit in avoiding elective inductions before 39 weeks' gestation (Main et al., 2011). Oregon, with leadership by the Oregon Perinatal Collaborative, is the first state to implement a "hard-stop policy" limiting elective inductions and cesarean deliveries before 39 weeks. This policy limits early-term deliveries by requiring review and approval by hospital OB/GYN departments for any delivery without documented indication before 39 weeks of gestation (Snowden et al., 2016).

Promoting Emotional Safety During Childbearing

Another factor that interrupts the physiologic process is the mother's perception of emotional safety. Any situation in which the mother feels threatened or unsupported can disturb pregnancy and birth. An example is the relived experience of sexual trauma. If all members of the healthcare team were educated to provide trauma-informed care, would they give thoughtful attention to protecting emotional safety during vaginal examinations?

There is solid scientific evidence that continuous support in labor promotes spontaneous vaginal birth, shorter duration of labor, and decreased caesarean or instrumental birth, use of any analgesia, use of regional anesthesia, and negative feelings about childbirth experiences (Bohren, Hofmeyr, Sakala, Fukuzawa, & Cuthbert, 2017). It also can protect emotional safety. While labor and delivery nurses or midwives usually provide excellent continuous labor support, inadequate staffing may make this impossible. Studies have shown that doulas serve well in this role (Bohren et al., 2017).

In the private pay health system in the United States, doulas are not generally available for underinsured women or for women on Medicaid for Pregnancy. Nationally, only 6% of women overall receive doula care (Childbirth

Connection, 2016). Two states, Minnesota and Oregon, have passed legislation that allows reimbursement for doula services for women on Medicaid (Association of State and Territorial Health Officials, 2018). Shafia Monroe, one of the contributors to this book, was one of the key leaders in this effort in Oregon (Waldroupe, 2012). Doula care shows promise for protecting emotional safety and promoting noninterventive outcomes, particularly for women at risk for racism (Kozhimannil, Hardeman, Attanasio, Blauer-Peterson, & O'Brien, 2013; Kozhimannil, Attanasio, et al., 2014; Kozhimannil et al., 2016). The Black Mamas Matter Alliance (blackmamasmatter.org), an advocacy group, is another group that is concerned with emotional safety. This organization reminds health providers that the traditional practices of many African Americans are a pathway to physiologic birth and emotional safety. Examples of traditional practices are family and doula involvement, midwifery care, food as medicine, and breastfeeding.

REDUCING CESAREAN BIRTH

The Prevalence and Risk of Cesarean Birth

There is widespread agreement that the cesarean birth rate has risen substantially and is too high. Cesarean increased from 22% to 33% of all births between 1998 and 2008 with a 50% increase among first births and a steep increase in subsequent births as vaginal birth after a prior cesarean became a concern (Barber et al., 2011; Main et al., 2011; Cunningham et al., 2010; Williams et al., 2018). The *Healthy People 2020* national goal for cesarean birth is 23.9% for low-risk first-time mothers (Healthy People 2020, n.d). A systematic review has shown that repeat cesarean carries a greater risk than vaginal birth after cesarean (VBAC) (Guise et al., 2010). The NIH consensus statement supported the safety of VBAC (Cunningham et al., 2010).

While cesarean can be a lifesaving procedure for mothers and babies, it is major abdominal surgery and the overall U.S. rate is twice the recommended level of the WHO (Lagrew et al., 2018). Across the nation, there is great variety in the rate. In 2017, the highest rates were in the Southern states, with Mississippi leading at 37.8%, and the lowest rates were in the West, with Utah leading at 22.5% (CDC, 2019).

In the Obstetric Care Consensus (2014), the ACOG and SMFM compared outcomes with vaginal and cesarean birth. Maternal mortality after cesarean is 3.7 times higher, amniotic fluid embolism is at least twice as high, and placental abnormalities increase with each subsequent cesarean birth (Caughey, Cahill, Guise, & Rouse, 2014).

The Systemic Factors Influencing Cesarean Birth

Unquestionably there are genuine, lifesaving reasons for cesarean, but in the United States much of the excess number of cesarean births closely track systemic factors in the healthcare delivery system.

Limited Access to Appropriate Level of Care

Cesarean rates are higher in rural areas (Menard et al., 2016). Nonmedically indicated primary cesarean as well as limited VBAC access is more common in rural, low-volume hospitals. These rates reflect a pragmatic and litigation-defensive solution to managing complications in areas of limited access to the appropriate level of care (Kozhimannil et al., 2015; Kozhimannil, Hung, et al., 2014; MacDorman & Declercq, 2016; Menard et al., 2016).

Provider Characteristics

Variability in provider has been shown to affect both primary and secondary cesarean rates. Obstetricians manage the highest risk patients, sometimes in a co-management relationship with midwives, but with ultimate responsibility for the patients at highest risk for cesarean. Surgeons and family practice physicians sometimes perform cesareans, especially in emergent or remote areas. While obstetricians generally are the providers to perform cesareans, there is great variability among obstetricians in the rate of cesareans. In rural areas, some family practice doctors are trained to do cesareans and on-call surgeons may be needed in the absence of other providers with this skill. The variability in cesarean rate is seen with both VBAC and primary (first-time) cesareans (Caughey et al., 2014). The prevention of cesarean is very important among low-risk, first-time mothers with a single fetus in a good birth position, known as "nulliparous, term, singleton, vertex" (NTSV; Caughey et al., 2014).

Midwifery care is protective against cesarean. The midwifery model of care focuses on management of low-risk women and continuous labor support (Loewenberg Weisband, Klebanoff, Gallo, Shoben, & Norris, 2018). As demonstrated in systematic review by the Cochrane Pregnancy and the Childbirth Group, both NTSV women and women seeking VBAC are more likely to have fewer interventions with midwifery births (Sandall, Soltani, Gates, Shennan, & Devane, 2016). Labor and delivery nurses have been shown to have both a positive and a negative impact on cesarean rate depending upon belief about the normalcy of birth, communication patterns with obstetricians, and the amount of continuous support during labor. This effect is seen particularly with primary cesarean among NTSV mothers (Edmonds, O'Hara, Clarke, & Shah, 2017).

Hospital Policies and Practices

The Leapfrog Group is a nonprofit organization that publishes public information data on cesarean rates voluntarily provided by hospitals. A 2015 Leapfrog Hospital Survey of 1,122 voluntary hospitals identified wide variety in hospital cesarean practices (Leapfrog Group, 2015). Kozhimannil, Law, and Virnig (2013) corroborated this finding identifying hospital rates of cesarean birth between 7.1% and 69.9% of births.

It has been established that African American mothers have disproportionate maternal mortality and morbidity, that cesarean birth carries a higher mortality and morbidity rate, and that Black mothers have higher cesarean rates compared to White mothers (Edmonds, Yehezkel, Liao, & Simas, 2013; Getahun et al., 2009; Howell, Egorova, Balbierz, Zeitlin, & Hebert, 2016). The question of whether there are different hospital practices based upon racial and ethnic profiles has been raised. In a large study of 1,475,457 births, maternal clinical diagnosis, including race and ethnicity, was compared to cesarean rates in 1,373 hospitals. There was a 25% spread in cesarean probability among institutions, pointing toward institutional factors (e.g., policies and established practices), rather than race or ethnicity, as decisive in the path toward cesarean (Kozhimannil, Arcaya, & Subramanian, 2014). In a multicenter study of 75,400 women, both NTSV and multiparas with prior vaginal births, Yee et al. (2017) found that Black NTSV women had a higher cesarean rate than White NTSV women, based upon clinical concern about fetal distress and failure to progress in labor (28.3% vs. 25%). Among multiparous women with prior vaginal births, only 6% had cesarean birth, more among Asian American women with provider concern about fetal distress. An interesting point is that the majority of these Asian American multiparous women with cesarean gave birth to an infant with a 1-minute Apgar of 7. These authors reported that they did not discover any evidence of differences in the provision of care associated with race or ethnicity (Yee et al., 2017).

A single institution-level study of 4,483 NTSV women demonstrated a difference in clinical decision making about fetal distress and failure to progress in labor by race and ethnicity. NTSV African American women, admitted for planned vaginal birth, had a disproportionally higher cesarean rate based upon subjective provider measures of fetal distress (Edmonds et al., 2013). Conversely, in large national studies in primarily White-serving hospitals, compared to primarily Black-serving hospitals, there were large differences in maternal outcome, including higher cesarean rates among Black mothers (Creanga et al., 2014; Howell et al., 2016). The findings raise the question of whether hospitals that serve primarily Black women differ in the definition of fetal distress or in provider understanding of fetal distress, based upon race. It also suggests that a focus on high risk among African American women may diminish attention to promoting physiologic birth.

Clinical Practices Addressing Social Determinants and Inequity in Cesarean Birth

Cesarean birth needs to be reserved as a lifesaving measure for mothers or babies. It carries surgical risk and is frequently performed on those who are most vulnerable by virtue of social determinants of health: poverty, geographical isolation, lack of access to healthcare, and racial and ethnic inequity. Some examples of clinical initiatives to decrease the cesarean rate are identified in Table 6.2. For instance, using

TABLE 6.2 Examples of Clinical Initiatives to Decrease the Cesarean Rate in the United States

INITIATIVE	ORGANIZATION	DESCRIPTION AND RESOURCES
Obstetric care consensus guidelines	American College of Obstetricians and Gynecologists (ACOG)/Society for Maternal-Fetal Medicine (SMFM) http://dx.doi.org/10.1016/j.ajog.2014.01.026	Specific guidelines, for example, promoting physiologic approach during first and second stage of labor, reposition of fetal occiput and version, enhanced skill with fetal heart monitoring, induction, and vaginal twin birth
Healthy birth initiative: Reducing primary cesareans	American College of Nurse-Midwives (ACNM) http://birthTOOLS.org/RPC-Learning-Collaborative	Multihospital learning collaborative to reduce NTSV through continuous labor support, increasing comfort in labor, and use of intermittent fetal heart auscultation
Reducing cesarean sections	The Leapfrog Group http://www.leapfroggroup.org	Educational materials for women Resources for providers Public information and dissemination of hospital cesarean rates
Cesarean deliveries, outcomes, and opportunities for change in California: Toward a public agenda for maternity care safety and quality	California Maternal Quality Care Collaborative (CMQCC) https://www.cmqcc.org/	CMQCC White Paper on Cesarean Deliveries
Safe reduction of primary cesarean births +AIM	Council on Patient Safety in Women's Health Care https://safehealthcareforeverywoman.org/patient-safety-bundles/safe-reduction-of-primary-cesarean-birth	Patient Safety Bundle with directions on readiness, recognition and prevention, response, and reporting systems for systems learning on safe reduction in cesarean birth Permission granted to disseminate
Strong start initiative for mothers and babies	Centers for Medicare and Medicaid Innovation and American Association of Birth Centers (AABC) http://www.birthcenters.org/?page=strongstart and http://www.birthcenters.org	Demonstration project in 45 AABC-accredited freestanding birth centers with enhanced care and peer counseling to reduce cesarean among Medicaid patients

NTSV, nulliparous, term, singleton, vertex.

guidelines from the Obstetric Care Consensus on not diagnosing labor arrest at 6 centimeters has decreased the cascade of events leading to cesarean (Caughey et al., 2014; Wilson-Leedy, DiSilvestro, Repke, & Pauli, 2016). The CMQCC Toolkit to Support Vaginal Birth and Reduce Primary Cesareans includes an implementation guide on averting this diagnosis (Smith, Peterson, Lagrew, & Main, 2017). Two maternal safety bundles that apply to cesarean birth in term of reducing inequity and promoting evidence-based practice are:

- Reduction of Peripartum Racial/Ethnic Disparities (+AIM) (ACOG, 2016b)
- Safe Reduction of Primary Cesarean Birth (+AIM) (ACOG, 2015c)

As of this writing, the new ARRIVE trial (Grobman et al., 2018) encouraging labor induction at 39 weeks as a means of reducing cesarean is controversial. There have been cautionary warnings by ACOG, ACNM, and CMQCC due to concern over reduction in physiologic birth and a potential rise in cesarean birth. (ACNM, 2018; ACOG, 2018; VanGompel et al., 2019)

PREVENTING AND MANAGING RISK

Care of childbearing women is centered on promoting normalcy, preventing adverse events, identifying risk, and managing risks if they arise. The CMQCC toolkits and the maternal safety bundles are designed to help providers and institutions provide consistent, evidence-based care. Yet, only about 40% of U.S. hospitals have adopted these toolkits and safety bundles (CBS News, 2018). Acceptance and implementation of these quality measures involve multiple levels of healthcare, including providers, managers, administrators, and oversight boards. A recent report on hospital governing board and management practices identified two critical factors characteristic of high-performing hospitals. The first factor was close board attention to the quality of clinical care. This oversight encouraged management staff to carefully monitor quality performance measures. The second factor was the utilization of clinical quality metrics in decision making by hospital governing boards. This practice encouraged management staff to set high-performance targets for improving delivery of care (Tsai et al., 2015). When quality measures are central to the discussion and decision making, then priority areas of maternal mortality and severe morbidity become more visible. The role of heart disease in maternal health is the prime example.

Awareness of Heart Disease

It may be counterintuitive to think of heart disease as the priority issue with young, apparently healthy pregnant women. Hypertension before and during the childbearing cycle doubles the risk of developing cardiovascular disease later in life

(Stuart et al., 2018) but it can also kill or maim during childbearing. Cardiovascular diseases, hypertensive disorders of pregnancy, and cardiomyopathy are the leading causes of death and disability during childbearing in the United States. Peripartum cardiomyopathy, sometimes asymptomatic until around 5 months postpartum, is linked to chronic hypertension, pregnancy-induced hypertension, and preeclampsia. African American women are disproportionally affected (Bello, Rendon, & Arany, 2013; Carlin, Alfirevic, & Gyte, 2010; Hilfiker-Kliner, Haghikia, Nonhoff, & Bauersachs, 2015; Irizarry et al., 2017).

Some of this pathology occurs before pregnancy, which underscores the importance of preconception care and expanded coverage under the Patient Protection and Affordable Care Act. However, pathology may also arise initially during the pregnancy or the postpartum. Providers need to focus on prevention, identification, and management of hypertension and cardiac or early preeclamptic signs during pregnancy. Often, swelling, shortness of breath, and fatigue are dismissed as normal pregnancy discomforts. Indeed, they may be. However, they can also be major warning signs of an impending cardiac or vascular event. Careful listening, observation, and rapid intervention are essential. Providers need to be ready to implement action as described in these patient safety bundles and toolkits:

- Severe Hypertension in Pregnancy (+AIM) (ACOG, 2015d)
- Maternal Early Warning Criteria (Council on Patient Safety in Women's Health Care, 2017)
- Reduction of Peripartum Racial/Ethnic Disparities (+AIM) (ACOG, 2016b)
- Support After a Severe Maternal Event (+AIM) (ACOG, 2015e)
- Improving Health Care Response to Cardiovascular Disease in Pregnancy and Postpartum (CMQCC, 2017)
- Improving Health Care Response to Preeclampsia (CMQCC, 2014)

Rising cardiac-related mortality and morbidity during childbearing is a harbinger of the social determinants of health. For instance, food security and adequate food during pregnancy is linked to cardiac health. Pregnant women with food insecurity who participate in food programs demonstrate better cardiovascular health (Morales, Epstein, Marable, Oo, & Berkowitz, 2016).

Alertness for Catastrophic Events

Most healthcare providers have high awareness of acute events such as obstetric hemorrhage, sepsis, thrombotic pulmonary embolism, or amniotic fluid embolism. However, a slow, insidious hemorrhage in a healthy, young woman may initially show subtle or no early vital sign changes. Embolism can also be slow to manifest. Both active listening to the mother and astute observation are essential clinical skills, as exemplified by the recent harrowing experience of tennis champion Serena Williams. (See Chapter 1.) Early warning systems help providers to have enhanced alertness to events that can quickly become catastrophic (Zuckerwise & Lipkind, 2017). The Maternal Early Warning Signs Protocol is an example of information that needs to be posted and readily available in all clinical settings (Council on Patient Safety in Women's Health Care, 2017). Team collaboration and well-defined algorithms are critical to rapid response, as described by the CMQCC Obstetric Quality Improvement Initiative (Bingham, Lyndon, Lagrew, & Main, 2011). Staff need to be well versed with the following safety bundles and toolkits:

- Obstetric Hemorrhage (+AIM) (ACOG, 2015b)

- Maternal Venous Thromboembolism (+AIM) (ACOG, 2015a)

- Maternal Early Warning Criteria (Council on Patient Safety in Women's Health Care, 2017)

- Reduction of Peripartum Racial/Ethnic Disparities (+AIM) (ACOG, 2016b)

- Support After a Severe Maternal Event (+AIM) (ACOG, 2015e)

- Improving Health Care Response to Obstetric Hemorrhage (CMQCC, 2015)

- Improving Health Care Response to Maternal Venous Thromboembolism (CMQCC, 2018)

Women with limited access to care are more likely to be at risk for catastrophic events during the childbearing cycle. Access to care is a social determinant of health. Timely and well-organized care and a well-prepared staff are essential components in preventing and managing catastrophic events.

Attentiveness to Life Course and Social Determinants of Mental Health

Among American mothers, maternal mortality related to suicide, homicide, and drug overdose is a strongly emerging trend, 16.2% of all late pregnancy-related deaths (Building U.S. Capacity, 2018). Intimate partner violence is implicated in over 54% of pregnancy-associated suicides, and among those childbearing women who are murdered, 45% involve intimate partner violence (Alhusen, Ray, Sharps, & Bullock, 2015; CDC, 2018; Palladino, Singh, Campbell, Flynn, & Gold, 2011; Wallace, Hoyert, Williams, & Mendola, 2016).

Screening pregnant women for these issues is evidence-based best practice. Sometimes, however, healthcare providers de facto blame the mother for her candor, either by verbal expressions or by the subtlest of nonverbal communication. Research shows that when the legal consequences of revealing these issues are high or the mother feels negated, she will deny or underreport these life stresses or even avoid healthcare altogether (Garg et al., 2016; Haycraft, 2018; Krans & Patrick, 2016). Is it any wonder that women hide information or avoid prenatal care when prior experience has shown them how harshly society views them, the potential for criminalization, and the limitations of available services?

Screening is only the first step. It lacks value unless there is action to address positive findings. Currently, community mental health services, shelters, and telehealth services are limited, especially for pregnant women in poverty (Andrulis, Siddiqui, Reddy, Jahnke, & Cooper, 2015; Smith, Johnson-Lawrence, Andrews, & Parker, 2017). Clinicians and mothers are often frustrated by this porous public health safety net. However, as providers view these adverse experiences nonjudgmentally through the paradigm of disrupting social determinants of health, pregnant women are more likely to feel listened to and helped, even in the face of scarce resources (Haycraft, 2018; Krans & Patrick, 2016). Referrals and interprofessional, collaborative initiatives are essential (Andrulis et al., 2015; Smith, Johnson-Lawrence, et al., 2017), but a warm, one-on-one relationship with the provider may be a lifeline.

Some patient safety bundles that can assist with guiding care and supporting mental health are:

- Maternal Mental Health: Depression and Anxiety (ACOG, 2016a)
- Obstetric Care for Women With Opioid Use Disorder (+AIM) (ACOG, 2017b)
- Postpartum Care Basics for Maternal Safety: Transition From Maternity to Well-Woman Care (+AIM) (ACOG, 2018a)
- Postpartum Care Basics for Maternal Safety: From Birth to the Comprehensive Postpartum Visit (+AIM) (ACOG, 2017c)
- Reduction of Peripartum Racial/Ethnic Disparities (+AIM) (ACOG, 2016b)
- Support After a Severe Maternal Event (+AIM) (ACOG, 2015e)

As mental health–related mortality occurs frequently in the postpartum, the patient safety bundles for postpartum transition are especially pertinent.

SUMMARY

Pregnancy-related morbidity and mortality is linked to racism and inequity embedded in the social determinants of health. Changing the paradigm in clinical care to one of equity requires consideration of the social determinants that shape the life course of a childbearing woman. It requires creating an evidence-based culture of safety that embraces equity, safeguards physiologic care, reduces unnecessary cesarean birth, and systematically prevents and manages risk.

WHAT IF

This section poses critical questions and discussion points about the crippling of health and the loss of life among America's mothers. It is an opportunity to think creatively about the issues of equity in maternal care. Consider the factors of racism and undermining social determinants as key factors affecting equity. Answers are deliberately not provided. The solutions to this national epidemic lie in interdisciplinary, imaginative conversation and problem solving. The authors invite the readers to consider these questions and add additional ones.

EQUITY IN CLINICAL CARE: ADDRESSING THE SOCIAL DETERMINANTS OF MATERNAL HEALTH

Discuss the *Healthy People 2020* focus on equity as the overarching goal for maternal health.

How would providing equity in healthcare impact social determinants of health?

Discuss patient safety bundles and toolkits in relation to increasing equity and access to care.

From a financial perspective, could doula support impact maternal outcomes?

Discuss the pros and cons of the cesarean epidemic in relation to the recent ARRIVE study promoting induction at 39 weeks. Why is this controversial from the perspective of providers, mothers, funders, and the community at large?

Describe the links between rising cardiac-related mortality and morbidity during childbearing and the social determinants of health. Compare this finding to the general health of the American population.

Discuss late postpartum mortality in relation to the social determinants of health.

REFERENCES

Agrawal, P. (2015). Maternal mortality and morbidity in the United States of America. *Bulletin of the World Health Organization, 93*(3), 135. doi:10.2471/BLT.14.148627

Alhusen, J., Ray, E., Sharps, P., & Bullock, L. (2015). Intimate partner violence during pregnancy: Maternal and neonatal outcomes. *Journal of Women's Health, 24*(1), 100–106. doi:10.1089/jwh.2014.4872

Alliance for Innovation on Maternal Health. (2015). AIM program fact sheet. Retrieved from   https://safehealthcareforeverywoman.org/wp-content/uploads/2016/10/AIM -Program-Fact-Sheet-v2.pdf

American College of Nurse-Midwives, Midwives Alliance North America, & National Association of Certified Professional Midwives. (2012). Supporting healthy and normal physiologic childbirth: A consensus statement by ACNM, MANA, and NACPM. Retrieved from http://www.midwife.org/ACNM/files/ACNMLibraryData/UPLOADFILENAME/000000000272/Physiological%20Birth%20Consensus%20Statement-%20FINAL%20May%2018%202012%20FINAL.pdf

American College of Nurse Midwives. (2018). Retrieved from http://www.midwife.org/ACNM-Responds-to-Release-of-ARRIVE-Trial-Study-Results

American College of Obstetricians and Gynecologists. (2015a). Maternal venous thromboembolism (+AIM). Retrieved from https://safehealthcareforeverywoman.org/patient-safety-bundles/maternal-venous-thromboembolism

American College of Obstetricians and Gynecologists. (2015b). Obstetric hemorrhage (+AIM). Retrieved from https://safehealthcareforeverywoman.org/patient-safety-bundles/obstetric-hemorrhage

American College of Obstetricians and Gynecologists. (2015c). Safe reduction of primary cesarean birth (+AIM). Retrieved from https://safehealthcareforeverywoman.org/patient-safety-bundles/safe-reduction-of-primary-cesarean-birth

American College of Obstetricians and Gynecologists. (2015d). Severe hypertension in pregnancy (+AIM). Retrieved from https://safehealthcareforeverywoman.org/patient-safety-bundles/severe-hypertension-in-pregnancy

American College of Obstetricians and Gynecologists. (2015e). Support after a severe maternal event (+AIM). Retrieved from https://safehealthcareforeverywoman.org/patient-safety-bundles/support-after-a-severe-maternal-event-supported-by-aim

American College of Obstetricians and Gynecologists. (2016a). Maternal mental health: Depression and anxiety. Retrieved from https://safehealthcareforeverywoman.org/patient-safety-bundles/maternal-mental-health-depression-and-anxiety

American College of Obstetricians and Gynecologists. (2016b). Reduction of peripartum racial/ethnic disparities (+AIM). Retrieved from https://safehealthcareforeverywoman.org/patient-safety-bundles/reduction-of-peripartum-racialethnic-disparities

American College of Obstetricians and Gynecologists. (2017a). Approaches to limit intervention during labor and birth (Committee Opinion No. 766). Retrieved from https://www.acog.org/Clinical-Guidance-and-Publications/Committee-Opinions/Committee-on-Obstetric-Practice/Approaches-to-Limit-Intervention-During-Labor-and-Birth

American College of Obstetricians and Gynecologists. (2017b). Obstetric care for women with opioid use disorder (+AIM). Retrieved from https://safehealthcareforeverywoman.org/patient-safety-bundles/obstetric-care-for-women-with-opioid-use-disorder

American College of Obstetricians and Gynecologists. (2017c). Postpartum care basics for maternal safety: From birth to the comprehensive postpartum visit (+AIM). Retrieved from https://safehealthcareforeverywoman.org/patient-safety-bundles/postpartum-care-basics-1

American College of Obstetricians and Gynecologists. (2018). Retrieved from https://www.acog.org/About-ACOG/News-Room/Statements/2018/ACOG-Response-to-ARRIVE-Trial?IsMobileSet=false

American College of Obstetricians and Gynecologists. (2018a). Postpartum care basics for maternal safety: Transition from maternity to well-woman care (+AIM). Retrieved from https://safehealthcareforeverywoman.org/patient-safety-bundles/postpartum-care-basics-2

American College of Obstetricians and Gynecologists. (2018b). Prevention of retained vaginal sponges after birth. Retrieved from https://safehealthcareforeverywoman.org/patient-safety-bundles/prevention-of-retained-vaginal-sponges

Amnesty International. (2011). *Deadly delivery: The maternal health care crisis in the USA: One-year update.* New York, NY: Amnesty International Publications. Retrieved from https://cdn2.sph.harvard.edu/wp-content/uploads/sites/32/2017/06/deadlydelivery oneyear.pdf

Andrulis, D., Siddiqui, N., Reddy, S., Jahnke, L., & Cooper, M. (2015). *Safety-net hospital systems transformation in the era of health care reform: Experiences, lessons, and perspectives from 13 safety-net systems across the nation.* Austin: Texas Health Institute. Retrieved from https://www.texashealthinstitute.org/uploads/1/3/5/3/13535548/safety-net_systems_transformation_in_era_of_reform_-_full_report.pdf

Association for Prevention Teaching and Research. (n.d.). Social determinants of health: Case studies. Retrieved from https://www.teachpopulationhealth.org/sdohcases.html

Association for Prevention Teaching and Research. (2018). Clinical prevention and population health in health professions education: Tackling the social determinants of health. Retrieved from https://health.gov/news/blog/2018/08/clinical-prevention-and-population-health-in-health-professions-education-tackling-the-social-determinants-of-health/?source=govd

Association of State and Territorial Health Officials. (2018). State policy approaches to incorporating doula services into maternal care [Blog post]. Retrieved from http://www.astho.org/StatePublicHealth/State-Policy-Approaches-to-Incorporating-Doula-Services-into-Maternal-Care/08-09-18

Bailit, J., Grobman, W., McGee, P., Reddy, U., Wapner, R., Varner, M., . . . Blackwell, S. (2015). Does the presence of a condition-specific obstetric protocol lead to detectable improvements in pregnancy outcomes? *American Journal of Obstetrics and Gynecology, 213*(1), 86.e1–86.e6. doi:10.1016/j.ajog.2015.01.055

Barber, E., Lundsberg, L., Belanger, K., Pettker, C., Funai, E., & Illuzzi, J. (2011). Indications contributing to the increasing cesarean delivery rate. *Obstetrics & Gynecology, 118*(1), 29–38. doi:10.1097/AOG.0b013e31821e5f65

Bello, N., Rendon, I., & Arany, Z. (2013). The relationship between pre-eclampsia and peripartum cardiomyopathy: A systematic review and meta-analysis. *Journal of the American College of Cardiology, 62*(18), 1715–1723. doi:10.1016/j.jacc.2013.08.717

Benfer, E. (2015). Health justice: A framework (and call to action) for the elimination of health inequity and social injustice. *The American University Law Review, 65*(2),

275–351. Retrieved from http://www.aulawreview.org/health-justice-a-framework-and-call-to-action-for-the-elimination-of-health-inequity-and-social-injustice

Bingham, D., Lyndon, A., Lagrew, D., & Main, E. (2011). A state-wide obstetric hemorrhage quality improvement initiative. *The American Journal of Maternal/Child Nursing, 36*(5), 297–304. doi:10.1097/NMC.0b013e318227c75f

Bohren, M., Hofmeyr, G., Sakala, C., Fukuzawa, R., & Cuthbert A. (2017). Continuous support for women during childbirth. *Cochrane Database of Systematic Reviews,* (7), CD003766. doi:10.1002/14651858.CD003766.pub6

Braveman, P., & Gottlieb, L. (2014). The social determinants of health: It's time to consider the causes of the causes. *Public Health Report, 129* (Suppl. 2), 19-31. doi:10.1177/003 33549141291S206

Building U.S. Capacity to Review and Prevent Maternal Deaths. (2018). *Report from nine maternal mortality review committees.* Retrieved from http://reviewtoaction.org/Report_from_Nine_MMRCs

Byhoff, E., Cohen, A., Hamati, M., Tatko, J., Davis, M., & Tipirneni, R. (2017). Screening for social determinants of health in Michigan Health Centers. *Journal of the American Board of Family Medicine, 30*(4), 418–427. doi:10.3122/jabfm.2017.04.170079

California Maternal Quality Care Collaborative. (n.d.-a). Toolkits. Retrieved from https://www.cmqcc.org/resources-tool-kits/toolkits

California Maternal Quality Care Collaborative. (n.d.-b). Who we are. Retrieved from https://www.cmqcc.org/who-we-are

California Maternal Quality Care Collaborative. (2014). Improving health care response to preeclampsia. Retrieved from https://www.cmqcc.org/resources-tool-kits/toolkits/preeclampsia-toolkit

California Maternal Quality Care Collaborative. (2015). Improving health care response to obstetric hemorrhage, v2.0. Retrieved from https://www.cmqcc.org/resources-tool-kits/toolkits/ob-hemorrhage-toolkit

California Maternal Quality Care Collaborative. (2017). Improving health care response to cardiovascular disease in pregnancy and postpartum. Retrieved from https://www.cmqcc.org/resources-toolkits/toolkits/improving-health-care-response-cardiovascular-disease-pregnancy-and

California Maternal Quality Care Collaborative. (2018). Improving health care response to maternal venous thromboembolism. Retrieved from https://www.cmqcc.org/resources-toolkits/toolkits/improving-health-care-response-maternal-venous-thromboembolism

Carlin, A., Alfirevic, Z., & Gyte, G. (2010). Interventions for treating peripartum cardiomyopathy to improve outcomes for women and babies. *Cochrane Database of Systematic Reviews,* (9). doi:10.1002/14651858.CD008589.pub2

Caughey, A. B., Cahill, A. G., Guise, J.-M., & Rouse, D. J. (2014). Safe prevention of the primary cesarean delivery. *American Journal of Obstetrics and Gynecology, 210*(3), 179–193. doi:10.1016/j.ajog.2014.01.026

CBS News. (2018, July 26). U.S. "most dangerous" place to give birth in developed world, USA Today investigation finds. Retrieved from https://www.cbsnews.com/news/us-most -dangerous-place-to-give-birth-in-developed-world-usa-today-investigation-finds

Centers for Disease Control and Prevention. (2010). *Selecting effective interventions.* Retrieved from https://www.cdc.gov/globalhealth/healthprotection/fetp/training_modules/ 7/selecting-interventions_pg_final_09252013.pdf

Centers for Disease Control and Prevention. (2018). *National vital statistics system, maternal mortality by State.* Retrieved from https://www.americashealthrankings.org/ explore/health-of-women-and-children/measure/maternal_mortality/state/ALL

Centers for Disease Control and Prevention. (2019). Cesarean delivery rate by state. Retrieved from https://www.cdc.gov/nchs/pressroom/sosmap/cesarean_births/cesareans.htm

Childbirth Connection. (2016). Overdue: Medicaid and private insurance coverage of doula care to strengthen maternal and infant health. Retrieved from http://www .nationalpartnership.org/research-library/maternal-health/overdue-medicaid-and -private-insurance-coverage-of-doula-care-to-strengthen-maternal-and-infant -health-issue-brief.pdf

Childbirth Connection. (2018). How do childbearing experiences differ across racial and ethnic groups in the United States? A *Listening to Mothers III* data brief. Retrieved from https://transform.childbirthconnection.org/reports/listeningtomothers/race-ethnicity

Council on Patient Safety in Women's Health Care. (n.d.). Patient safety bundles. Retrieved from https://safehealthcareforeverywoman.org/patient-safety-bundles

Council on Patient Safety in Women's Health Care. (2017). Maternal early warning criteria. Retrieved from https://safehealthcareforeverywoman.org/patient-safety-tools/ maternal-early-warning-criteria

Creanga, A., Bateman, B., Mhyre, J., Kuklina, E., Shilkrut, A., & Callaghan, W. (2014). Performance of racial and ethnic minority-serving hospitals on delivery-related indicators. *American Journal of Obstetrics and Gynecology, 211*(6), 647.e1–647.e16. doi:10.1016/j.ajog.2014.06.006

Cunningham, F. G., Bangdiwala, S., Brown, S. S., Dean, T. M., Frederiksen, M., Rowland Hogue, C. J., . . . Zimmet, S. C. (2010). *National Institutes of Health consensus development conference statement: Vaginal birth after cesarean: New insights.* Retrieved from http://consensus.nih.gov/2010/images/vbac/vbac_statement.pdf

D'Angelo, K., Bryan, J., & Kurz, B. (2015). Women's experiences with prenatal care: A mixed-methods study exploring the influence of the social determinants of health. *Journal of Health Disparities Research and Practice, 9*(3), 9. Retrieved from https:// digitalscholarship.unlv.edu/jhdrp/vol9/iss3/9

Declercq, E., Sakala, C., Corry, M., Applebaum, S., & Herrlich, A. (2013). *Listening to mothers III: Pregnancy and birth.* Retrieved from http://www.nationalpartnership.org/re search-library/maternal-health/listening-to-mothers-iii-pregnancy-and-birth-2013.pdf

Division for Heart Disease and Stroke Prevention. (n.d.). Healthy People 2020. Retrieved from https://www.cdc.gov/dhdsp/hp2020.htm

Edmonds, B., Mogul, M., & Shea, J. (2015). Understanding low-income African American women's expectations, preferences, and priorities in prenatal care. *Family and Community Health, 38*(2), 149–157. doi:10.1097/FCH.0000000000000066

Edmonds, J., O'Hara, M., Clarke, S., & Shah, N. (2017). Variation in cesarean birth rates by labor and delivery nurses. *Journal of Obstetric, Gynecologic & Neonatal Nursing, 46*(4), 486–493. doi:10.1016/j.jogn.2017.03.009

Edmonds, J., Yehezkel, R., Liao, X., & Simas, T. (2013). Racial and ethnic differences in primary unscheduled cesarean deliveries among low-risk primiparous women at an academic medical center: A retrospective study. *BMC Pregnancy and Childbirth, 13,* 168. Retrieved from http://www.biomedcentral.com/1471-2393/13/168

Gadson, A., Akpovi, E., & Mehta, P. (2017). Exploring the social determinants of racial/ethnic disparities in prenatal care utilization and maternal outcome. *Seminars in Perinatology, 41*(5), 308–317. doi:10.1053/j.semperi.2017.04.008

Gany, F., Lee, T., Ramirez, J., Massie, D., Moran, A., Crist, M., . . . Leng, J. (2014). Do our patients have enough to eat? Food insecurity among urban low-income cancer patients. *Journal of Health Care for the Poor and Underserved, 25*(3), 1153–1168. doi:10.1353/hpu.2014.0145

Garg, M., Garrison, L., Leeman, L., Hamidovic, A., Borrego, M., Rayburn, W., & Bakhireva, L. (2016). Validity of self-reported drug use information among pregnant women. *Maternal and Child Health Journal, 20*(1), 41–47. doi:10.1007/s10995-015-1799-6

Getahun, D., Strickland, D., Lawrence, J., Fassett, M., Koebnick, C., & Jacobsen, S. (2009). Racial and ethnic disparities in the trends in primary cesarean delivery based on indications. *American Journal of Obstetrics and Gynecology, 201*(4), 422.e1–422.e7. doi:10.1016/j.ajog.2009.07.062

Grobman, W., Rice, M., Reddy, U., Tita, A., Silver, R., Mallett, G., . . . Macones, G. A. (2018). Labor induction versus expectant management in low-risk nulliparous women. *New England Journal of Medicine, 379,* 513–523. doi:10.1056/NEJMoa1800566

Guise, J., Eden, K., Emeis, C., Denman, M., Marshall, N., Fu, R., . . . McDonagh, M. (2010). *Vaginal birth after cesarean: New insights* (Evidence Report/Technology Assessment No. 191, AHRQ Publication No. 10-E003). Rockville, MD: Agency for Healthcare Research and Quality.

Haberkorn, J. (2018, August 22). Maternal mortality rates in the U.S. have risen steadily. Sen. Kamala Harris has a plan to change that. *Los Angeles Times.* Retrieved from https://www.latimes.com/politics/la-na-pol-congress-harris-maternal-health-20180822-story.html

Hardeman, R., Medina, E., & Kozhimannil, K. (2016). Structural racism and supporting Black lives—The role of health professionals. *New England Journal of Medicine, 375*(22), 2113–2115. doi:10.1056/NEJMp1609535

Haycraft, A. (2018). Pregnancy and the opioid epidemic. *Journal of Psychosocial Nursing and Mental Health Services, 56*(3), 19–23. doi:10.3928/02793695-20180219-03

Healthy People 2020. (n.d.). *Maternal, Infant, and Child Health, Morbidity and Mortality Objective MICH-7.1.* Retrieved from https://www.healthypeople.gov/2020/topics-objectives/topic/maternal-infant-and-child-health/objectives

Hilfiker-Kleiner, D., Haghikia, A., Nonhoff, J., & Bauersachs, J. (2015). Peripartum cardio-myopathy: Current management and future perspectives. *European Heart Journal*, *36*(18), 1090–1097. doi:10.1093/eurheartj/ehv009

Hoffman, K., Trawalter, S., Axt, J., & Oliver, M. (2016). Racial bias in pain assessment and treatment recommendations, and false beliefs about biological differences between Blacks and Whites. *Proceedings of the National Academy of Sciences of the United States of America, 113*(16), 4296–4301. doi:10.1073/pnas.1516047113

Howell, E., Egorova, N., Balbierz, A., Zeitlin, J., & Hebert, P. (2016). Black-White differences in severe maternal morbidity and site of care. *American Journal of Obstetrics and Gynecology, 214*(1), 122.e1–122.e7. doi:10.1016/j.ajog.2015.08.019

Hughes, L. (2016). Social determinants of health and primary care: Intentionality is key to the data we collect and the interventions we pursue. *Journal of the American Board of Family Medicine, 29*(3), 297–300. doi:10.3122/jabfm.2016.03.160120

Institute for Healthcare Improvement. (n.d.). What is a bundle? Retrieved from http://www.ihi.org/resources/Pages/ImprovementStories/WhatIsaBundle.aspx

Institute of Medicine. (2011). *The future of nursing: Leading change, advancing health.* Washington, DC: National Academies Press. Retrieved from http://www.nap.edu/catalog.php?record_id=12956

Interprofessional Education Collaborative Expert Panel. (2011). *Core competencies for interprofessional collaborative practice: Report of an expert panel.* Washington, DC: Interprofessional Education Collaborative. Retrieved from https://www.aacom.org/docs/default-source/insideome/ccrpt05-10-11.pdf?sfvrsn=77937f97_2

Irizarry, O., Levine, L., Lewey, J., Boyer, T., Riis, V., Elovitz, M., & Arany, Z. (2017). Comparison of clinical characteristics and outcomes of peripartum cardiomyopathy between African American and non–African American Women. *JAMA Cardiology, 2*(11), 1256–1260. doi:10.1001/jamacardio.2017.3574

Kaplan, K., Mestel, P., & Feldman, D. (2010). Creating a culture of mutual respect. *AORN Journal, 91*(4), 495–510. doi:10.1016/j.aorn.2009.09.031

King, T., & Pinger, W. (2014). Evidence-based practice for intrapartum care: The pearls of midwifery. *Journal of Midwifery and Women's Health, 59*(6), 572–585. doi:10.1111/jmwh.12261

Kozhimannil, K., Arcaya, M., & Subramanian, S. (2014). Maternal clinical diagnosis and hospital variation in the risk of cesarean delivery: Analyses of a national US hospital discharge database. *PLOS Medicine, 11*, e1001745. doi:10.1371/journal.pmed.1001745

Kozhimannil, K., Attanasio, L., Jou, J., Joarnt, L., Johnson, P., & Gjerdingen, D. (2014). Potential benefits of increased access to doula support during childbirth. *American Journal of Managed Care, 20*(8), e340–e352. Retrieved from https://www.ajmc.com/journals/issue/2014/2014-vol20-n8/potential-benefits-of-increased-access-to-doula-support-during-childbirth

Kozhimannil, K., Casey, M., Hung, P., Han, X., Prasad, S., & Moscovice, I. (2015). The rural obstetric workforce in US hospitals: Challenges and opportunities. *Journal of Rural Health, 31*(4), 365–372. doi:10.1111/jrh.12112

Kozhimannil, K., Hardeman, R., Attanasio, L., Blauer-Peterson, C., & O'Brien, M. (2013). Doula care, birth outcomes, and costs among Medicaid beneficiaries. *American Journal of Public Health, 103*(4), e113–e121. doi:10.2105/AJPH.2012.301201

Kozhimannil, K., Hung, P., Prasad, S., Casey, M., McClellan, M., & Moscovice, I. (2014). Birth volume and the quality of obstetric care in rural hospitals. *Journal of Rural Health, 30*(4), 335–342. doi:10.1111/jrh.12061

Kozhimannil, K., Law, M., & Virnig, B. (2013). Cesarean delivery rates vary tenfold among US hospitals; reducing variation may address quality and cost issues. *Health Affairs, 32*(3), 527–535. doi:10.1377/hlthaff.2012.1030

Kozhimannil, K., Vogelsang, C., Hardeman, R., & Prasad, S. (2016). Disrupting the pathways of social determinants of health: Doula support during pregnancy and childbirth. *Journal of the American Board of Family Medicine, 29*(3), 308–317. doi:10.3122/jabfm.2016.03.150300

Krans, E., & Patrick, S. (2016). Opioid use disorder in pregnancy: Health policy and practice in the midst of an epidemic. *Obstetrics & Gynecology, 128*(1), 4–10. doi:10.1097/AOG.0000000000001446

Lagrew, D. C., Low, L. K., Brennan, R., Corry, M., Edmonds, J., Gilpin, B. G., . . . Jaffer, S. (2018). National partnership for maternal safety: Consensus bundle on safe reduction of primary cesarean births—Supporting intended vaginal births. *Obstetrics & Gynecology, 131*(3), 503–513. doi:10.1097/AOG.0000000000002471

The Leapfrog Group. (2015). *C-section rates by hospital.* Retrieved from http://www.leapfroggroup.org/ratings-reports/rate-c-sections

Loewenberg Weisband, Y., Klebanoff, M., Gallo, M., Shoben, A., & Norris, A. (2018). Birth outcomes of women using a midwife versus women using a physician for prenatal care. *Journal of Midwifery and Women's Health, 63*(4), 399–409. doi:10.1111/jmwh.12750

MacDorman, M., & Declercq, E. (2016). Trends and characteristics of United States out-of-hospital births 2004–2014: New information on risk status and access to care. *Birth, 43*(2), 116–124. doi:10.1111/birt.12228

Main, E., Morton, C., Hopkins, D., Giuliani, G., Melsop, K., & Gould, J. (2011). Cesarean deliveries, outcomes, and opportunities for change in California: Toward a public agenda for maternity care safety and quality. Retrieved from https://www.cmqcc.org/resource/cesarean-deliveries-outcomes-and-opportunities-change-california-toward-public-agenda

Main, E., Oshiro, B., Chagolla, B., Bingham, D., Dang-Kilduff, L., & Kowalewski, L. (2010). *Elimination of non-medically indicated (elective) deliveries before 39 weeks gestational age.* Palo Alto: California Maternal Quality Care Collaborative. Retrieved from https://health.usf.edu/publichealth/chiles/fpqc/~/media/41ACFEE060F24D2AB70295BAF4221889.ashx

Mazul, M., Salm Ward, T., & Ngui, E. (2017). Anatomy of good prenatal care: Perspectives of low income African-American women on barriers and facilitators to prenatal care.

Journal of Racial and Ethnic Health Disparities, 4(1), 79–86. doi:10.1007/s40615-015 -0204-x

Menard, K., Kilpatrick, S., Saade, G., Hollier, L., Joseph, G., Jr., Barfield, W., . . . Conry, J. (2015). Levels of maternal care. *American Journal of Obstetrics and Gynecology, 212*(3), 259–271. doi:10.1016/j.ajog.2014.12.030

Morales, M., Epstein, M., Marable, D., Oo, S., & Berkowitz, S. (2016). Food insecurity and cardiovascular health in pregnant women: Results from the Food for Families Program, Chelsea, Massachusetts, 2013–2015. *Preventing Chronic Disease, 13*, 160212. doi:10.5888/pcd13.160212

National Conference of State Legislatures. (2011). Healthy People 2020 and maternal and child health. Retrieved from http://www.ncsl.org/research/health/healthy-people-2020-and-maternal-and-child-health.aspx#maternal

Office of Disease Prevention and Health Promotion. (n.d.). Disparities. Retrieved from https:// www.healthypeople.gov/2020/about/foundation-health-measures/Disparities#5

Palladino, C., Singh, V., Campbell, J., Flynn, H., & Gold, K. (2011). Homicide and suicide during the perinatal period: Findings from the National Violent Death Reporting System. *Obstetrics & Gynecology, 118*(5), 1056–1063. doi:10.1097/AOG.0b013e 31823294da

Rawls, J. (1971). *A theory of justice*. Cambridge, MA: Harvard University Press.

Reeves, S., Perrier., Goldman, J., Feeth, D., & Zwarenstein, M. (2013). Interprofessional education: Effects on professional practice and healthcare outcomes (update). *The Cochrane Database of Systematic Reviews*, (3), CD002213. doi:10.1002/14651858 .CD002213.pub3

Sakara, C., Romano, A., & Buckley, S. (2016). Hormonal physiology of childbearing, an essential framework for maternal-newborn nursing. *Journal of Obstetric, Gynecologic, & Neonatal Nursing, 45*(2), 264–275. doi:10.1016/j.jogn.2015.12.006

Sandall, J., Soltani, H., Gates, S., Shennan, A., & Devane, D. (2016). Midwife-led continuity models versus other models of care for childbearing women. *Cochrane Database of Systematic Reviews*, (4), CD004667. doi:10.1002/14651858.CD004667.pub5

Smith, L., Johnson-Lawrence, V., Andrews, M., & Parker, S. (2017). Opportunity for interprofessional collaborative care—Findings from a sample of federally qualified health center patients in the Midwest. *Public Health, 151*, 131–136. doi:10.1016/j .puhe.2017.07.009

Smith, H., Peterson, N., Lagrew, D., & Main, E. (2017). Toolkit to support vaginal birth and reduce primary cesareans. Retrieved from https://www.cmqcc.org/VBirthToolkit

Snowden, J., Muoto, I., Darney, B., Quigley, B., Tomlinson, M., Neilson, D., . . . Caughey, A. (2016). Oregon's hard-stop policy limiting elective early-term deliveries: Association with obstetric procedure use and health outcomes. *Obstetrics & Gynecology, 128*(6): 1389–1396. doi:10.1097/AOG.0000000000001737

Stuart, J., Tanz, L., Missmer, S., Rimm, E., Spiegelman, D., James-Todd, T., & Rich-Edwards, J. (2018). Hypertensive disorders of pregnancy and maternal cardiovascular disease risk factor development: An observational cohort study. *Annals of Internal Medicine, 169*(4), 224–232. doi:10.7326/M17-2740

Tsai, T., Jha, A., Gawande, A., Huckman, R., Bloom, N., & Sadun, R. (2015). Hospital board and management practices are strongly related to hospital performance on clinical quality metrics. *Health Affairs, 34*(8), 1304–1311. doi:10.1377/hlthaff.2014.1282

VanGompel, E. W., Perez, S., Datta, A., Wang, C., Cape, V., & Main, E. (2019). Cesarean overuse and the culture of care. *Health Services Research, 54*(2), 417–424. doi:10.1111/1475-6773.13123

Waldroupe, A. (2012). Workgroup recommends Oregon health plan use doulas. *The Lund Report.* Retrieved from https://www.thelundreport.org/content/workgroup-recommends-oregon-health-plan-use-doulas

Wallace, M., Hoyert, D., Williams, C., & Mendola, P. (2016). Pregnancy-associated homicide and suicide in 37 US states with enhanced pregnancy surveillance. *American Journal of Obstetrics and Gynecology, 215*(3), 364.e1–364.e10. doi:10.1016/j.ajog.2016.03.040

Williams, C., Asaolu, I., Chavan, N., Williamson, L., Lewis, A., Beaven, L., & Ashford, K. (2018). Previous cesarean delivery associated with subsequent preterm birth in the United States. *European Journal of Obstetrics and Gynecology and Reproductive Biology, 229*, 88–93. doi:10.1016/j.ejogrb.2018.08.013

Williams, D. (2016). How racism makes us sick. *TED Talk.* Retrieved from https://www.ted.com/talks/david_r_williams_how_racism_makes_us_sick?utm_source=tedcomshare&utm_medium=email&utm_campaign=tedspread

Wilson-Leedy, J., DiSilvestro, A., Repke, J., & Pauli, J. (2016) Reduction in the cesarean delivery rate after obstetric care consensus guideline implementation. *Obstetrics & Gynecology, 128*(1), 145–152. doi:10.1097/AOG.0000000000001488

Woolf, S., & Aron, L. (Eds.). (2013). *U.S. health in international perspective: Shorter lives, poorer health.* Washington, DC: National Academies Press.

Yee, L., Costantine, M., Rice, M., Bailit, J., Reddy, U., Wapner, R., . . . Tolosa, J. (2017). Racial and ethnic differences in utilization of labor management strategies intended to reduce cesarean delivery rates. *Obstetrics & Gynecology, 130*(6), 1285–1294. doi:10.1097/AOG.0000000000002343

Yongue, C. M., Caiola, C., & Dixon, C. (2017). Seeking health equity: Examining racism as a social determinant of health. Retrieved from https://www.teachpopulationhealth.org/racismsdohcases.html

Zuckerwise, L., & Lipkind, H. (2017). Maternal early warning systems—Towards reducing preventable maternal mortality and severe maternal morbidity through improved clinical surveillance and responsiveness. *Seminars in Perinatology, 41*(3), 161–165. doi:10.1053/j.semperi.2017.03.005

PUBLIC HEALTH SERVICES

A Porous Safety Net

LISA R. ROBERTS

At the end of this chapter, the reader will be able to:

1. Describe the current status of the public health safety net in the United States.

2. Identify gaps in the public health safety net affecting maternal health.

3. Discuss policy that undermines the safety net for maternal health.

THE CURRENT SAFETY NET IN THE UNITED STATES

The public health safety net is a complex web of healthcare systems and programs that protects the health of Americans (Andrulis, Siddiqui, Reddy, Jahnke, & Cooper, 2015). The term "safety net" is typically used to describe public health services provided for both the general population and those with vulnerability. Vulnerable persons have increased claim on basic health services, preventive screening, and social support such as food and housing programs (Sufrin, 2017). The public health safety net for vulnerable mothers includes:

- Social services for housing

- Food programs

- Transportation services

- Medicaid for pregnancy

- Patient Protection and Affordable Care Act (ACA)

- Federally qualified healthcare centers (FQHCs)

- Mental health services

- Legal aid
- Criminal justice services

Social Services for Housing

Adequate housing is an important support for maternal health. Data over the last decade indicate a rise in women and children who are homeless in the United States. Among homeless women, almost 30% are of childbearing age. Homeless women or those with unstable living conditions (e.g., transient arrangements or motels) are at increased risk for:

- Violence
- Chronic physical conditions
- Mental health problems
- Substance abuse
- Difficulty managing weight (Cutts et al., 2015)

These risk factors are increased in combination (Cutts et al., 2015). Low-income women at particular risk for homelessness need availability of low-cost housing (Hinshaw, 2017). The U.S. government has tried to address homelessness through legislation and budgeting for the United States Interagency Council on Homelessness (USICH) and the American Recovery and Reinvestment Act of 2009. The goal is to prevent homelessness, or assist with rapid rehousing, rather than relying on emergency shelters and transitional housing. Additionally, temporary housing programs, shelters, and low-cost housing funded by federal or state government and nonprofit organizations supplement the safety net for housing (Cutts et al., 2015; Hinshaw, 2017).

Food Programs

Food insecurity, which affects as much as 33% of the general population, is higher among pregnant women (David, 2017; Morales, Epstein, Marable, Oo, & Berkowitz, 2016). It is associated with gestational diabetes, hypertension, anemia, and poor birth outcomes, making food security programs critical for maternal health. These safety net resources include the Supplemental Nutrition Assistance Program (SNAP; previously known as the "food stamp program"), the Special Supplemental Nutrition Program for Women, Infants, and Children (WIC), and local food banks. Eligibility requirements for these programs differ. SNAP requires verification of income at the poverty level (David, 2017). WIC serves low-income women who are pregnant and up to 6-weeks postpartum (U.S. Department of Agriculture, 2018). Food banks generally serve the local indigent population. Pregnant women with food insecurity who participate in food programs demonstrate better cardiovascular health (Morales et al., 2016).

Transportation Services

Transportation services vary tremendously across the nation. The use of public transportation has increased by 30% since 1995 (American Public Transportation Association, n.d.). Women with access to transportation are more likely to enter prenatal care early and consistently attend prenatal and postnatal appointments (Downe, Finlayson, Tunçalp, & Gülmezoglu, 2016).

Medicaid

Medicaid, serving primarily low-income persons, pays for almost half of all births in the United States (Markus, Krohe, Garro, Gerstein, & Pellegrini, 2017). Among women who delay prenatal care, 40% report lack of insurance or financial stress as the reason (Health Resources and Services Administration [HRSA], 2013). Women are often first enrolled in Medicaid when pregnant. Federal law requires that states taking part in the Medicaid program must provide coverage for poor pregnant women whether or not they are employed. However, women on the edge of poverty are frequently excluded from Medicaid due to restrictive income eligibility (Markus, Andres, West, Garro, & Pellegrini, 2013).

The ACA

The ACA expands coverage and access for maternal healthcare (Agrawal, 2015; Patient Protection and Affordable Care Act, 2010). The expansion of Medicaid coverage with the ACA offers primary care for prepregnancy and comorbid conditions during pregnancy (Bello, Rendon, & Arany, 2013; Creanga & Callaghan, 2017; Creanga et al., 2015; Florio, Daming, & Grodzinsky, 2018; Metcalfe, Wick, & Ronksley, 2018).

Federally Qualified Healthcare Centers

FQHCs are an important part of the public health safety net, sometimes partnering with or taking the place of local health departments (Snider, Bekemeier, Conrad, & Grembowski, 2017). Local health departments continue to be an important safety net for basic prenatal care, often when FQHCs are in the same geographical area (Snider et al., 2017). FQHCs, however, provide critical access to care for low-income mothers with higher than average risk for chronic disease (Jacobson et al., 2016; Smith, Johnson-Lawrence, Andrews, & Parker, 2017). Otherwise, these women may not receive risk-appropriate prenatal care (Snider et al., 2017). Of special concern are cardiovascular diseases as they are the leading cause of maternal mortality (Bello et al., 2013). Pregnant women in rural areas are particularly dependent on FQHCs as they are more likely to have limited, late-entry prenatal care and travel long distances for care (Jacobson et al., 2016). In states where FQHCs have adopted the ACA expansion to Medicaid, the quality of care has improved (Cole, Galárraga, Wilson, Wright, & Trivedi, 2017).

Access to care is not the only barrier for rural women. Rural women may face lack of choice or cultural mismatch with providers, poverty, poor health status, and high risk for substance abuse, mental health issues, and intimate partner violence (IPV; Douthit, Kiv, Dwolatzky, & Biswas, 2015). For all of these reasons, Medicaid enhancement with ACA coverage at FQHCs is an essential part of the public health safety net.

Mental Health Services

Women with high levels of stress and comorbid depression are more likely to become pregnant unintentionally than those without these issues (Hall, Kusunoki, Gatny, & Barber, 2014). Childbearing women may experience perinatal anxiety, depression, perinatal mental health complications, and postpartum psychosis (O'Hara & Wisner, 2014). FQHCs offer limited mental health services (Smith, Johnson-Lawrence, et al., 2017). Interprofessional, collaborative initiatives can improve mental health, quality of life, and the safety net (Smith, Johnson-Lawrence, et al., 2017), especially if offered in the medical-home model of care (Andrulis et al., 2015).

Legal Aid and Criminal Justice Services

Legal aid services address the social determinants of health. The assistance of civil attorney and legal aid services is vital for low-income women of childbearing age. Prior and current life course factors, such as poverty, affect health at the time of pregnancy (Atkins, Heller, DeBartolo, & Sandel, 2014). Pregnant women are at increased risk for IPV with poor health outcomes (Bermele, Andresen, & Urbanski, 2018). While few women experiencing IPV actually seek legal services (arrest or restraining order), those who take this step usually experience reduced abuse and decreased vulnerability. The 1994 Violence Against Women Act (VAWA), credited with 53% decrease in IPV in the United States between 1993 and 2008 (Ellsberg et al., 2015), is part of the public health safety net.

GAPS IN THE SAFETY NET
Social Services Gaps

There are significant gaps in the public health safety net, including housing, transportation, and water safety. Social services for housing are inadequate (Hinshaw, 2017). Data from studies over the last decade indicate that 4% to 9% of prenatal women experience homelessness (Cutts et al., 2015). Homeless women or those in transient housing such as shelters also have limited access to adequate nutrition and ability to prepare food (Cutts et al., 2015). Food insecurity is experienced by up to 11% of women during pregnancy (David, 2017; Morales et al., 2016; Sorensen,

Murray, Lemery, & Balbus, 2018). In spite of the SNAP (food stamp) program and WIC, food insecurity is a persistent issue in the United States (David, 2017).

Public transportation services are limited across most of the nation. Most people rely on private automobiles. Outside of a few major metropolitan areas, many cities lack adequate public transportation. It is estimated that 45% of the U.S. population does not have access to public transportation of any kind. Many residents of rural areas may have no access to transportation at all (American Public Transportation Association, n.d.; Burnett et al., 2016). Maternal health services are usually provided in centralized locations with the trend toward decreasing availability in rural areas (Downe et al., 2016; Sofer, 2017). Transportation issues and poverty limit the ability to keep appointments for care (Douthit et al., 2015; Downe et al., 2016; Edmonds, Mogul, & Shea, 2015).

Another aspect of the public health safety net is safe drinking water. Chemical contamination in public water supplies does occur (Quansah et al., 2015; Schade et al., 2015; Stacy et al., 2015). Pregnant women, fearing unsafe drinking water, may drink less or be dependent upon expensive bottled water, putting them at risk for dehydration. Dehydration during pregnancy is serious, as it decreases uterine blood flow and increases the risk for preterm labor (Schade et al., 2015; Sorensen et al., 2018). Drinking water contaminated with arsenic, often found in rural wells, is associated with increased risk of anemia during pregnancy, postpartum hypertension, and perinatal loss (Quansah et al., 2015). When water supply is compromised, the safety net has failed.

Healthcare Coverage Gaps

Despite Medicaid with ACA expansion, pregnant women often delay prenatal care while waiting for Medicaid coverage to begin (D'Angelo, Bryan, & Kurz, 2016; Edmonds et al., 2015). FQHCs and local health departments are overcrowded and do not have the capacity to fully meet the health needs of poor mothers. Limited budgets, politics, and changing priorities in healthcare contribute to diminished services provided by local health departments. Collaborations between some local health departments and FQHCs do not always succeed in providing full coverage (Snider et al., 2017). As a result, low-income pregnant women frequently seek unscheduled, hospital-based care (Mehta, Carter, Vinoya, Kangovi, & Srinivas, 2017).

Mental Health Services Gaps

Mental health and behavioral disorders contribute to disability among childbearing women (Baron et al., 2016). Women with a history of mental health issues or IPV have increased risk for perinatal mood and anxiety disorders (PMAD). These disorders affect 15% to 21% of childbearing women. Other contributing risk factors are limited education, poor social support, perinatal loss, or preterm birth (Byrnes, 2018; Hutti et al., 2018). Low-income pregnant women are less likely to receive mental health services than those with more resources (Bledsoe et al., 2017). The closure of state-run mental hospitals in the 1960–70s created demand for community-based mental health services. However, community services and programs with interdisciplinary teams or telehealth at FQHCs and Level 1 hospitals are limited (Andrulis et al., 2015; Smith, Johnson-Lawrence, et al., 2017).

Treatment facilities for drug-addicted pregnant women are also limited. Over-prescription of high-dose opioids, even after normal vaginal delivery, feeds into the opioid epidemic (Prabhu et al., 2018; Terplan, Longinaker, & Appel, 2015). Drug addiction and mental illness create a cyclical pattern of incarceration (Sufrin, 2017).

Legal Aid and Criminal Justice Services Gaps

The criminal justice system often fails to protect these high-risk mothers. Due to insufficient funding and staffing, legal aid clinics are overstretched (Atkins et al., 2014). Drug-addicted mothers often do not receive legal aid services in a timely manner, or at all (Ellsberg et al., 2015; Messing, O'Sullivan, Cavanaugh, Webster, & Campbell, 2017; Sufrin, 2017). Women make up 9% of the U.S. incarcerated population of which 5.5% are childbearing age. Among women of childbearing age in jail or prison, an estimated 6% to 10% are pregnant. They often receive inadequate or no prenatal care at all (Bard, Knight, & Plugge, 2016; Goshin, Arditti, Dallaire, Shlafer, & Hollihan, 2017; Maruschak, 2018; Sufrin, 2017).

The high incarceration rate of women, including pregnant mothers, related to drug offenses and homelessness, raises the issue of the criminalization of poverty (Sufrin, 2017; United Nations Human Rights Council [UNHRC], 2018). No national oversight or accrediting bodies ensure that correctional facilities comply with recommended professional standards of care (Cardaci, 2013). The United States does not meet the international human rights standards for pregnant incarcerated women (Goshin et al., 2017; UNHRC, 2018).

POLICIES AFFECTING THE SAFETY NET

Changes to national policies, such as the ACA inclusion of maternal care as an essential health benefit, were forecasted to improve maternal health outcomes (Agrawal, 2015). However, some recent policy changes have eroded the public health safety net for mothers (see Table 7.1).

Welfare Reform

The Personal Responsibility and Work Opportunity Reconciliation Act of 1996 (PRWORA, 1996), also known as "welfare reform," decreased economic dependence but has also had some negative consequences. Many low-income mothers are not able to afford health insurance or healthcare despite joining the workforce (Basu, Rehkopf, Siddiqi, Glymour, & Kawachi, 2016). Other women decline resources

TABLE 7.1 Examples of Policies Affecting the Public Health Safety Net for Maternal Health

POLICIES	POSITIVE AND NEGATIVE IMPACTS ON SAFETY NET	REFERENCES
Welfare Reform –PRWORA	Decreased dependence on social services Low-paying jobs with limited healthcare affordability Income scrutiny for requested services Lack of data on extent of non-governmental safety net services provided in communities	Basu et al., 2016 Hughes, 2018
Access to Reproductive Health Services – ACA – Contraception –Therapeutic abortion – Funded preventive care services (STIs, breast care, Pap smears)	Increased prepregnancy coverage and enhanced coverage with Medicaid Decreased individual ability to plan timing for healthy pregnancy Decreased to no availability especially in rural areas Decreased availability especially for low-income women	Cartwright et al., 2018 Guttmacher Institute, 2018 Molina & Pace, 2017 Richards, 2018 Stevenson et al., 2016 Maternal Mortality and Morbidity Task Force & Texas Department of State Health Services, 2019
Place-of-Birth Choice – ACA – Access to freestanding birth centers	Enhanced birth center coverage with Medicaid Failure to subscribe to ACA limits choice on safe, low-cost community-based birth and expanded choice of providers	AABC, 2015 Alliman et al., 2015 Cole & Avery, 2017 Edmonds et al., 2015 Smith, Gifford, et al., 2017 Stone, Ernst, & Stapleton, 2017 Torio & Moore, 2016
Family and Medical Leave	Federal mandate is *unpaid* family leave *Paid* leave by private employers results in longer maternity leaves, reduced medical costs, less absenteeism, and lower subsequent unemployment rates	Neckermann, 2017 Plotka & Busch-Rossnagel, 2018 Schönberg & Ludsteck, 2014
Reversal of Climate Change Policies	Failure to address climate change consequences and epidemic impacts, for example, Zika virus	Sorensen et al., 2018

AABC, American Association of Birth Centers; ACA, Patient Protection and Affordable Care Act; PRWORA, Personal Responsibility and Work Opportunity Reconciliation Act; STI, sexually transmitted infection.

fearing intrusive scrutiny. Some prefer to use resources provided by nonprofit organizations, including churches (Hughes, 2018). Unless data on utilization are shared, planning for an adequate public health safety net is difficult.

Reproductive Health Choice

Reproductive choices are restricted, especially in rural areas. Recent changes in national- or state-level policy have affected access to contraception, legal abortion, screening, and the treatment of reproductive health conditions (e.g., sexually transmitted infections [STIs], breast care, and Pap smears; Cartwright, Karunaratne, Barr-Walker, Johns, & Upadhyay, 2018; Molina & Pace, 2017). For instance, in 2011, the Texas State Legislature cut two thirds of the budget for state-level reproductive health services, forcing 80 clinics to shut down and effectively eliminating access to care for many women (Maternal Mortality and Morbidity Task Force & Texas Department of State Health Services, 2019; Reddan, 2016; Stevenson, Flores-Vazquez, Allgeyer, Schenkkan, & Potter, 2016).

Between 2011 and 2014, the number of legal abortion sites in the United States decreased by about 50%. By 2014, the legal abortion rate in the United States had decreased by 12% to 14.6/1,000 women aged 15 to 44, the lowest rate since abortion was legalized in 1973. Between 1998 and 2010, however, 20% of these legal abortions were medically indicated due to severe medical conditions with high risk of maternal mortality (Guttmacher Institute, 2018). At the time of this writing, there are increasing numbers of nonlicensed, community-based organizations and Internet sites advertising "do-it-yourself" abortion as well as non-evidence-based information on the risks of abortion versus pregnancy.

In some states, restriction on medication-induced abortion leaves higher risk surgical abortion as the only legal option. Medication restriction, as opposed to surgical abortion, is not evidence based but rather is a political choice, increasing risk for women choosing legal abortion. Restricting Planned Parenthood affiliations from using public funds to provide healthcare services may have been intended to curb legal abortion rates in the United States, but it has also significantly affected women's contraceptive choices and access to reproductive healthcare (Richards, 2018). Decreased contraceptive availability results in unplanned pregnancies and increased Medicaid coverage for births (Stevenson et al., 2016).

Place of Birth

Policy also affects choice for place of birth. The majority of states recognize birth centers and most private insurers cover the costs (Alliman, Jolles, & Summers, 2015; American Association of Birth Centers [AABC], 2015). Some states, however, have declined to participate in the ACA, which supplements birth center costs under Medicaid (Stone, Ernst, & Stapleton, 2017). Since Medicaid covers the cost of nearly 50% of births in the United States (Smith, Gifford, et al., 2017; Torio & Moore, 2016) but insufficiently covers birth center costs without ACA enhancement, this policy effectively eliminates freestanding birth centers as a choice for many women (Cole & Avery, 2017; Edmonds et al., 2015). Many women have expressed preference for the midwifery model of care in birth centers, but if they are funded by Medicaid alone, birth centers may not be able to meet expenses (Cole & Avery, 2017; Edmonds et al., 2015).

Family and Medical Leave

The 1993 Family and Medical Leave Act (FMLA) mandates that employers provide *unpaid* maternity leave of 12 weeks. However, many women do not benefit from this policy due to exceptions for small businesses and part-time employees (Neckermann, 2017; Schönberg & Ludsteck, 2014). The length of maternity leave varies tremendously due to lack of a federal policy for *paid* maternity leave. The idea of paid leave is controversial, although it is normative in most developed nations. Paid leave encourages mothers to take longer maternity leaves. The outcomes are reduced medical costs, less absenteeism, and lower unemployment rates (Plotka & Busch-Rossnagel, 2018; Schönberg & Ludsteck, 2014).

California earned an A rating for leading the way with the first paid family leave law in the nation, providing employees with 55% of their wages for up to 6 weeks. California remains the best-rated state for maternity leave with an increase to 70% of wages paid in 2018. On the opposite coast, New York and Washington, DC, have the next highest ratings. New York earned an A- for a step-wise plan to increase paid leave to 12 weeks by 2021, and DC also earned an A-. Twelve states are rated as the worst for maternity leave, earning less than C ratings because they have not passed any new laws protecting mothers since FMLA was enacted (Huang & Yang, 2015).

Reversal of Climate Change Policies

Policies that inhibit measures to address climate change affect maternal health. For instance, rising temperatures, decreased rain and water supplies, and altered ecology change geographical distribution of vector-borne and waterborne illnesses. Emergence of the Zika epidemic is an example. Pregnant women are more susceptible to vector-borne and waterborne illnesses and have more severe illnesses than nonpregnant women, increasing risk for maternal morbidity and mortality (Sorensen et al., 2018).

SUMMARY

The maternal mortality crisis in the United States stems, in part, from policies that have shaped the current U.S. healthcare system. Reducing pregnancy-related morbidity and mortality involves not only providing clinical care but addressing disparities in policy and in the public health safety net (Bingham, Suplee, Morris, & McBride, 2018). Recently the U.S. Senate proposed $50 million in new funding to address maternal mortality. The stated intention for the funding is maternal mortality prevention. The Centers for Disease Control and Prevention (CDC) would receive 24% of funds to expand data collection and research on maternal morbidity and mortality and to guide state-level morbidity and mortality review boards. The Maternal and Child Health Bureau would be allocated 76% of the money to provide support for evidence-based efforts to improve maternal health, primarily through the Alliance for Innovation on Maternal Health (AIM) and Healthy Start programs (Martin, 2018; see also https://safehealthcareforeverywoman.org/aim-program and https://mchb.hrsa.gov/sites/default/files/mchb/MaternalChildHealthInitiatives/healthy-start-infographic.pdf.)

Healthy Start is a very worthy project, focusing on many aspects of maternal and child health. The challenge will be to keep a tight focus on maternal health to ensure that maternal health is not defined in terms of the "other," lost in the policy shuffle of multiple national needs. As Kate Womersley, the producer of the National Public Radio (NPR) media series *Lost Mothers*, points out, the mother is still perceived as a vessel for the unborn child rather than a full partner in the dyad of new life (Womersley, 2017). Much work remains to mend the porous public health safety net for maternal health.

WHAT IF

This section poses critical questions and discussion points about the crippling of health and the loss of life among America's mothers. It is an opportunity to think creatively about the public health safety net. Answers are deliberately not provided. The solutions to this national epidemic lie in interdisciplinary, imaginative conversation and problem solving. The authors invite the readers to consider these questions and add additional ones.

PUBLIC HEALTH SERVICES: A POROUS SAFETY NET

What forms of technology can develop safety net patches in areas of high need?

How would decriminalizing addiction and not treating poverty as a crime improve maternal health?

What would be the impact of national legislation mandating paid maternity leave?

What are the implications for the safety net and for low-income women if the ACA is weakened in scope for provision of both primary care and funding of birth centers?

Discuss the interface of restrictions on climate change policies and the health of pregnant women.

Evaluate the downstream effects of decreasing or eliminating Planned Parenthood funding for low-income women.

REFERENCES

Agrawal, P. (2015). Maternal mortality and morbidity in the United States of America. *Bulletin of the World Health Organization, 93*(3), 135. doi:10.2471/BLT.14.148627

Alliman, J., Jolles, D., & Summers, L. (2015). The innovation imperative: Scaling freestanding birth centers, CenteringPregnancy, and midwifery-led maternity health homes. *Journal of Midwifery and Women's Health, 60*(3), 244–249. doi:10.1111/jmwh.12320

American Association of Birth Centers. (2015). Update on AABC Medicaid survey of birth centers. *AABC News.* Retrieved from https://www.birthcenters.org/store/ViewProduct.aspx?ID=10046031

American Public Transportation Association. (n.d.). Facts. Retrieved from https://www.apta.com/mediacenter/ptbenefits/Pages/FactSheet.aspx

Andrulis, D., Siddiqui, N., Reddy, S., Jahnke, L., & Cooper, M. (2015). *Safety-net hospital systems transformation in the era of health care reform: Experiences, lessons, and perspectives from 13 safety-net systems across the nation.* Austin: Texas Health Institute. Retrieved from https://www.texashealthinstitute.org/uploads/1/3/5/3/13535548/safety-net_systems_transformation_in_era_of_reform_-_executive_summary.pdf

Atkins, D., Heller, S., DeBartolo, E., & Sandel, M. (2014). Medical-legal partnership and Healthy Start: Integrating civil legal aid services into public health advocacy. *Journal of Legal Medicine, 35*(1), 195–209. doi:10.1080/01947648.2014.885333

Bard, E., Knight, M., & Plugge, E. (2016). Perinatal health care services for imprisoned pregnant women and associated outcomes: A systematic review. *BMC Pregnancy and Childbirth, 16*(1), 285. doi:10.1186/s12884-016-1080-z

Baron, E., Hanlon, C., Mall, S., Honikman, S., Breuer, E., Kathree, T., ... Tomlinson, M. (2016). Maternal mental health in primary care in five low- and middle-income countries: A situational analysis. *BMC Health Services Research, 16*(1), 53. doi:10.1186/s12913-016-1291-z

Basu, S., Rehkopf, D., Siddiqi, A., Glymour, M., & Kawachi, I. (2016). Health behaviors, mental health, and health care utilization among single mothers after welfare reforms in the 1990s. *American Journal of Epidemiology, 183*(6), 531–538. doi:10.1093/aje/kwv249

Bello, N., Rendon, I., & Arany, Z. (2013). The relationship between pre-eclampsia and peripartum cardiomyopathy: A systematic review and meta-analysis. *Journal of the American College of Cardiology, 62*(18), 1715–1723. doi:10.1016/j.jacc.2013.08.717

Bermele, C., Andresen, P., & Urbanski, S. (2018). Educating nurses to screen and intervene for intimate partner violence during pregnancy. *Nursing for Women's Health, 22*(1), 79–86. doi:10.1016/j.nwh.2017.12.006

Bingham, D., Suplee, P., Morris, M., & McBride, M. (2018). Healthcare strategies for reducing pregnancy-related morbidity and mortality in the postpartum period. *The Journal of Perinatal and Neonatal Nursing, 32*(3), 241–249. doi:10.1097/JPN.0000000000000344

Bledsoe, S., Rizo, C., Wike, T., Killian-Farrell, C., Wessel, J., Bellows, A., & Doernberg, A. (2017). Pregnant adolescent women's perceptions of depression and psychiatric services in the United States. *Women and Birth, 30*(5), e248–e257. doi:10.1016/j.wombi.2017.02.006

Burnett, C., Schminkey, D., Milburn, J., Kastello, J., Bullock, L., Campbell, J., & Sharps, P. (2016). Negotiating peril: The lived experience of rural, low-income women exposed to IPV during pregnancy and postpartum. *Violence Against Women, 22*(8), 943–965. doi:10.1177/1077801215614972

Byrnes, L. (2018). Perinatal mood and anxiety disorders. *The Journal for Nurse Practitioners, 14*(7), 507–513. doi:10.1016/j.nurpra.2018.03.010

Cardaci, R. (2013). Care of pregnant women in the criminal justice system. *American Journal of Nursing, 113*(9), 40–48. doi:10.1097/01.NAJ.0000434171.38503.77

Cartwright, A., Karunaratne, M., Barr-Walker, J., Johns, N., & Upadhyay, U. (2018). Identifying national availability of abortion care and distance from major US cities: Systematic online search. *Journal of Medical Internet Research, 20*(5), e186. doi:10.2196/jmir.9717

Cole, L., & Avery, M. (Eds.). (2017). *Freestanding birth centers: Innovation, evidence, optimal outcomes.* New York, NY: Springer Publishing Company.

Cole, M., Galárraga, O., Wilson, I., Wright, B., & Trivedi, A. (2017). At federally funded health centers, Medicaid expansion was associated with improved quality of care. *Health Affairs, 36*(1), 40–48. doi:10.1377/hlthaff.2016.0804

Creanga, A., & Callaghan, W. (2017). Recent increases in the U.S. maternal mortality rate: Disentangling trends from measurement issues. *Obstetrics & Gynecology, 129*(1), 206–207. doi:10.1097/AOG.0000000000001831

Creanga, A., Berg, C., Syverson, C., Seed, K., Bruce, F., & Callaghan, W. (2015). Pregnancy-related mortality in the United States, 2006–2010. *Obstetrics & Gynecology, 125*(1), 5–12. doi:10.1097/AOG.0000000000000564

Cutts, D., Coleman, S., Black, M., Chilton, M., Cook, J., Ettinger de Cuba, S., . . . Frank, D. (2015). Homelessness during pregnancy: A unique, time-dependent risk factor of birth outcomes. *Maternal and Child Health Journal, 19*(6), 1276–1283. doi:10.1007/s10995-014-1633-6

D'Angelo, K., Bryan, J., & Kurz, B. (2016). Women's experiences with prenatal care: A mixed-methods study exploring the influence of the social determinants of health. *Journal of Health Disparities Research and Practice, 9*(3), 9. Retrieved from https://digitalscholarship.unlv.edu/jhdrp/vol9/iss3/9

David, E. (2017). *Food insecurity in America: Putting dignity and respect at the forefront of food aid. Samuel Centre for Social Connectedness: Social Connectedness Fellowship Program.* Retrieved from http://www.socialconnectedness.org/wp-content/uploads/2018/02/Food-Insecurity-in-America-Putting-Dignity-and-Respect-at-the-Forefront-of-Food-Aid.pdf

Douthit, N., Kiv, S., Dwolatzky, T., & Biswas, S. (2015). Exposing some important barriers to health care access in the rural USA. *Public Health, 129*(6), 611–620. doi:10.1016/j.puhe.2015.04.001

Downe, S., Finlayson, K., Tunçalp, Ö., & Gülmezoglu, A. (2016, October 20). Factors that influence the uptake of routine antenatal services by pregnant women: A qualitative evidence synthesis. *The Cochrane Database of Systematic Reviews, 2016*(10), CD012392. doi:10.1002/14651858.CD012392

Edmonds, B., Mogul, M., & Shea, J. (2015). Understanding low-income African American women's expectations, preferences, and priorities in prenatal care. *Family & Community Health, 38*(2), 149–157. doi:10.1097/FCH.0000000000000066

Ellsberg, M., Arango, D., Morton, M., Gennari, F., Kiplesund, S., Contreras, M., & Watts, C. (2015). Prevention of violence against women and girls: What does the evidence say? *The Lancet, 385*(9977), 1555–1566. doi:10.1016/S0140-6736(14)61703-7

Florio, K., Daming, T., & Grodzinsky, A. (2018). Poorly understood maternal risks of pregnancy in women with heart disease. *Circulation, 137*(8), 766–768. doi:10.1161/CIR CULATIONAHA.117.031889

Goshin, L., Arditti, J., Dallaire, D., Shlafer, R., & Hollihan, A. (2017). An international human rights perspective on maternal criminal justice involvement in the United States. *Psychology, Public Policy, and Law, 23*(1), 53–67. doi:10.1037/law0000101

Guttmacher Institute. (2018). *Induced abortion in the United States.* New York, NY: Guttmacher Institute. Retrieved from https://www.guttmacher.org/fact-sheet/induced -abortion-united-states

Hall, K., Kusunoki, Y., Gatny, H., & Barber, J. (2014). The risk of unintended pregnancy among young women with mental health symptoms. *Social Science & Medicine, 100*, 62–71. doi:10.1016/j.socscimed.2013.10.037

Health Resources and Services Administration. (2013). *Child Health USA 2013.* Retrieved from: https://mchb.hrsa.gov/chusa13/dl/pdf/chusa13.pdf

Hinshaw, R. (2017). *The unsheltered woman: Women and housing.* New York, NY: Routledge. Retrieved from https://www.taylorfrancis.com/books/e/9781351302197

Huang, R., & Yang, M. (2015). Paid maternity leave and breastfeeding practice before and after California's implementation of the nation's first paid family leave program. *Economics & Human Biology, 16*, 45–59. doi:10.1016/j.ehb.2013.12.009

Hughes, C. (2018, June 29). From the long arm of the state to eyes on the street: How poor African American mothers navigate surveillance in the social safety net. *Journal of Contemporary Ethnography.* Advance online publication. doi:10.1177/089124161 8784151

Hutti, M., Myers, J., Hall, L., Polivka, B., White, S., Hill, J., . . . Kloenne, E. (2018). Predicting need for follow-up due to severe anxiety and depression symptoms after perinatal loss. *Journal of Obstetric, Gynecologic & Neonatal Nursing, 47*(2), 125–136. doi:10.1016/j.jogn.2018.01.003

Jacobson, L., Duong, J., Grainger, D., Collins, T., Farley, D., Wolfe, M., . . . Anderson B. (2016). Health assessment of a rural obstetrical population in a Midwestern state. *Journal of Pregnancy and Child Health, 3*, 252. doi:10.4172/2376-127X.1000252

Markus, A. R., Andres, E., West, K. D., Garro, N., & Pellegrini, C. (2013). Medicaid covered births, 2008 through 2010, in the context of the implementation of health reform. *Women's Health Issues, 23*(5), e273–e280. doi:10.1016/j.whi.2013.06.006

Markus, A. R., Krohe, S., Garro, N., Gerstein, M., & Pellegrini, C. (2017). Examining the association between Medicaid coverage and preterm births using 2010–2013 National Vital Statistics Birth Data. *Journal of Children and Poverty, 23*(1), 79–94. doi:10.1080/10796126.2016.1254601

Martin, N. (2018, June 28). U.S. Senate committee proposes $50 million to prevent mothers dying in childbirth. *ProPublica.* Retrieved from https://www.propublica.org/article/us-senate-committee-maternal-mortality-prevention-proposal

Maruschak, L. (2018, July 20). *Medical problems of prisoners* [Press release]. Retrieved from https://www.bjs.gov/content/pub/html/mpp/mpp.cfm

Maternal Mortality and Morbidity Task Force & Texas Department of State Health Services. (2019). Retrieved from https://www.dshs.texas.gov/mch/maternal_mortality_and_morbidity.shtm

Mehta, P., Carter, T., Vinoya, C., Kangovi, S., & Srinivas, S. (2017). Understanding high utilization of unscheduled care in pregnant women of low socioeconomic status. *Women's Health Issues, 27*(4), 441–448. doi:10.1016/j.whi.2017.01.007

Messing, J., O'Sullivan, C., Cavanaugh, C., Webster, D., & Campbell, J. (2017). Are abused women's protective actions associated with reduced threats, stalking, and violence perpetrated by their male intimate partners? *Violence Against Women, 23*(3), 263–286. doi:10.1177/1077801216640381

Metcalfe, A., Wick, J., & Ronksley, P. (2018). Racial disparities in comorbidity and severe maternal morbidity/mortality in the United States: An analysis of temporal trends. *Acta Obstetricia et Gynecologica Scandinavica, 97*(1), 89–96. doi:10.1111/aogs.13245

Molina, R., & Pace, L. (2017). A renewed focus on maternal health in the United States. *New England Journal of Medicine, 377*(18), 1705–1707. doi:10.1056/NEJMp1709473

Morales, M., Epstein, M., Marable, D., Oo, S., & Berkowitz, S. (2016). Food insecurity and cardiovascular health in pregnant women: Results from the Food for Families Program, Chelsea, Massachusetts, 2013–2015. *Preventing Chronic Disease, 13*, 160212. doi:10.5888/pcd13.160212

Neckermann, C. (2017). An international embarrassment: The United States as an anomaly in maternity leave policy. *Harvard International Review, 38*(3), 36–39. Retrieved from http://hir.harvard.edu/archive/?s=Christina%20Neckermann

O'Hara, M., & Wisner, K. (2014). Perinatal mental illness: Definition, description and aetiology. *Best Practice & Research Clinical Obstetrics & Gynaecology, 28*(1), 3–12. doi:10.1016/j.bpobgyn.2013.09.002

Patient Protection and Affordable Care Act, 42 U.S.C. § 18001 et seq. (2010).

Personal Responsibility and Work Opportunity Reconciliation Act, Pub. L. No. 104-193, sec. 103 (1996).

Plotka, R., & Busch-Rossnagel, N. A. (2018). The role of length of maternity leave in supporting mother–child interactions and attachment security among American mothers and their infants. *International Journal of Child Care and Education Policy, 12*(1), 2. doi:10.1186/s40723-018-0041-6

Prabhu, M., Garry, E., Hernandez-Diaz, S., MacDonald, S., Huybrechts, K., & Bateman, B. (2018). Frequency of opioid dispensing after vaginal delivery. *Obstetrics & Gynecology, 132*(2), 459–465. doi:10.1097/AOG.0000000000002741

Quansah, R., Armah, F., Essumang, D., Luginaah, I., Clarke, E., Marfoh, K., . . . Dzodzomenyo, M. (2015). Association of arsenic with adverse pregnancy outcomes/infant mortality: A systematic review and meta-analysis. *Environmental Health Perspectives, 123*(5), 412–421. doi:10.1289/ehp.1307894

Reddan, M. (2016). Texas has highest maternal mortality rate in developed world, study finds. *The Guardian.* Retrieved from https://www.theguardian.com/us-news/2016/aug/20/texas-maternal-mortality-rate-health-clinics-funding

Richards, C. (2018). *Make trouble: Standing up, speaking out, and finding the courage to lead—My life story.* New York, NY: Simon & Schuster.

Schade, C., Wright, N., Gupta, R., Latif, D., Jha, A., & Robinson, J. (2015). Self-reported household impacts of large-scale chemical contamination of the public water supply, Charleston, West Virginia, USA. *PLoS ONE, 10*(5), e0126744. doi:10.1371/journal.pone.0126744

Schönberg, U., & Ludsteck, J. (2014). Expansions in maternity leave coverage and mothers' labor market outcomes after childbirth. *Journal of Labor Economics, 32*(3), 469–505. doi:10.1086/675078

Smith, L., Johnson-Lawrence, V., Andrews, M., & Parker, S. (2017). Opportunity for interprofessional collaborative care—Findings from a sample of federally qualified health center patients in the Midwest. *Public Health, 151,* 131–136. doi:10.1016/j.puhe.2017.07.009

Smith, V., Gifford, K., Ellis, E., Edwards, B., Rudowitz, R., Hinton, E., . . . Valentine, A. (2017). *Implementing coverage and payment initiatives: Results from a 50-state Medicaid budget survey for state fiscal years 2016 and 2017.* Retrieved from https://www.kff.org/medicaid/report/implementing-coverage-and-payment-initiatives-results-from-a-50-state-medicaid-budget-survey-for-state-fiscal-years-2016-and-2017

Snider, J., Bekemeier, B., Conrad, D., & Grembowski, D. (2017). Federally qualified health center substitution of local health department services. *American Journal of Preventive Medicine, 53*(4), 405–411. doi:10.1016/j.amepre.2017.06.006

Sofer, D. (2017). Women in rural America are losing hospital-based obstetric services. *American Journal of Nursing, 117*(12), 14–15. doi:10.1097/01.NAJ.0000527469.46588.dc

Sorensen, C., Murray, V., Lemery, J., & Balbus, J. (2018). Climate change and women's health: Impacts and policy directions. *PLOS Medicine, 15*(7), e1002603. doi:10.1371/journal.pmed.1002603

Stacy, S., Brink, L., Larkin, J., Sadovsky, Y., Goldstein, B., Pitt, B., & Talbott, E. (2015). Perinatal outcomes and unconventional natural gas operations in Southwest Pennsylvania. *PLoS ONE, 10*(6), e0126425. doi:10.1371/journal.pone.0126425

Stevenson, A., Flores-Vazquez, I., Allgeyer, R., Schenkkan, P., & Potter, J. (2016). Effect of removal of Planned Parenthood from the Texas Women's Health Program. *New England Journal of Medicine, 374*(9), 853–860. doi:10.1056/NEJMsa1511902

Stone, S. E., Ernst, E. K. M., & Stapleton, S. R. (2017). The freestanding birth center: Evidence for change in the delivery of health care to childbearing families. In B. Anderson, J. Rooks, & R. Barroso (Eds.), *Best practices in midwifery: Using the evidence to implement change* (2nd ed., pp. 261–281). New York, NY: Springer Publishing Company.

Sufrin, C. (2017). *Jailcare: Finding the safety net for women behind bars*. Oakland: University of California Press.

Terplan, M., Longinaker, N., & Appel, L. (2015). Women-centered drug treatment services and need in the United States, 2002–2009. *American Journal of Public Health, 105*(11), e50–e54. doi:10.2105/AJPH.2015.302821

Torio, C., & Moore, B. (2016). *National inpatient hospital costs: The most expensive conditions by payer, 2013* (Statistical Brief #204). Rockville, MD: Agency for Healthcare Research and Quality. Retrieved from https://www.hcup-us.ahrq.gov/reports/statbriefs/sb204-Most-Expensive-Hospital-Conditions.jsp

United Nations Human Rights Council. (2018). *Report of the Special Rapporteur on extreme poverty and human rights on his mission to the United States of America*. Retrieved from https://digitallibrary.un.org/record/1629536/files/A_HRC_38_33_Add-1-EN.pdf

U.S. Department of Agriculture. (2018). WIC eligibility requirements. Retrieved from https://www.fns.usda.gov/wic/wic-eligibility-requirements

Womersley, K. (2017). Lost mothers: Why giving birth is safer in Britain than in the U.S. Retrieved from https://www.propublica.org/article/why-giving-birth-is-safer-in-britain-than-in-the-u-s

MENDING THE MATERNAL HEALTH SAFETY NET

Community-Based Strategies

BARBARA A. ANDERSON | JOYCE M. KNESTRICK

OBJECTIVES

At the end of this chapter, the reader will be able to:

1. Describe strategies to improve accuracy in obtaining, analyzing, and disseminating data on maternal mortality and severe morbidity in the United States.

2. Identify community-based innovations to improve the maternal health safety net.

3. Discuss educational initiatives to promote equity and life course management.

MENDING THE SAFETY NET

The World Health Organization (WHO) links escalating maternal mortality and morbidity in the United States to poor data quality, lack of standardized care, and/or delayed recognition in obstetric emergencies and a fragmented network of services and access to care (Agrawal, 2015). Maternal mortality and morbidity reflect the landscape in America: pervasive undermining social conditions; structural and systemic forces controlling access to services; and policies that have shaped inequity in healthcare. Reducing pregnancy-related mortality and severe morbidity requires equity in clinical care and improved access to the public health safety net (Bingham, Suplee, Morris, & McBride, 2018).

The discussion on maternal health has frequently been lost in the shuffle of multiple public health needs. A tight focus on promoting maternal health is essential to resolve issues of incomplete data, fragmentation of the safety net, and inattention to destructive social variables that define the life course for many childbearing women. This chapter examines efforts to improve the quality of data, presents exemplars of community-based innovations, and discusses school-based health education using life course theory as strategies to strengthen the maternal health safety net.

IMPROVING THE DATA

Official maternal mortality data are collected by the National Vital Statistics System, the Pregnancy Mortality Surveillance System, and state-level maternal mortality review committees (MMRCs; St. Pierre, Zaharatos, Goodman, & Callaghan, 2018). However, the United States lacks systematic data collection or consistent analysis of maternal mortality or severe morbidity. Many states lack maternal mortality review boards (WHO, United Nations International Children's Emergency Fund, United Nations Population Fund, World Bank Group, & United Nations Population Division, 2015). In addition, widely different time frames are used to define maternal mortality, crippling data comparison across states or internationally (MacDorman, Declercq, Cabral, & Morton, 2016). Standardized and shared data using common terminology as well as state and local maternity review boards could become the most efficient means of obtaining data (St. Pierre et al., 2018).

The public is slowly becoming aware of this issue due to reports from Amnesty International, the United Nations Humans Rights Council, National Public Radio, and *USA Today*. Recently, *USA Today* reported that at least 30 states have failed to review maternal deaths or have not investigated the healthcare delivered. Among the 10 states with the highest death rates, only four examined issues of care (Ungar, 2018). As of this writing, there is a proposed national-level funding at both Senate and House of Representative levels to enable the Centers for Disease Control and Prevention (CDC) to guide states in the development and refinement of maternal mortality review boards.

CDC Building Capacity Project

The CDC has taken the leadership in developing the Maternal Mortality Review Data System (MMRDS) and the Maternal Mortality Review Information Application (MMRIA) through a nine-state initiative representing 92% of U.S. maternal deaths (Building U.S. Capacity to Review and Prevent Maternal Deaths, 2018). The nine participating states in this project are Colorardo, Delaware, Georgia, Hawaii, Illinois, North Carolina, Ohio, South Carolina, and Utah.

The report from this project identifies six key decisions that an MMRC should make with each death review. These decisions are:

- Was the death pregnancy-related?
- What was the underlying cause of death?
- Was the death preventable?

- What were the factors that contributed to the death?

- What are the recommendations and actions that address those contributing factors?

- What is the anticipated impact of those actions if implemented? (Building U.S. Capacity, 2018, p. 10)

Contributing factors to the death are defined across five domains (community, facility, provider, patient/family, and systems of care) with a scoring rubric to help review committees target the key contributing factors by cause of death (Building U.S. Capacity, 2018). For instance, key contributing factors with hemorrhage are generally provider and systems of care, pointing to the need for ongoing provider education, readiness response teams, system access, and use of the safety bundles in standardizing care. Each of the six decisions has supporting material to help the MMRC analyze, document, and capture the data (Building U.S. Capacity, 2018). Systematic and consistent analysis of the causes and the cascade of events leading to each maternal death can provide data in developing road maps for clinical care and public health safety nets.

Severe Maternal Morbidity Institutional Review Panels

Data on severe maternal morbidity (SMM) are collected using the following methods: disease-specific condition; specified intervention; and organ-system dysfunction criteria (Creanga et al., 2014). SMM, often life threatening, is much more prevalent than maternal death. It affects an estimated 50,000 to 60,000 women each year and is increasing (CDC, 2017a, 2017b; Chen, Chauhan, & Blackwell, 2018; Creanga et al., 2014; Howell, Egorova, Balbierz, Zeitlin, & Hebert, 2016). Like maternal mortality, tracking SMM lacks systematic and continuous data collection (Agrawal, 2015; Creanga et al., 2014). Review of SMM events may not occur at the institution level, and if they do, the methods of data collection may not adequately assess the level of acuity, the extent of lifesaving intervention required, or the time frame for recovery.

Patient safety toolkits have been developed to help institutions systematically analyze SMM. These toolkits have been vetted by the Alliance for Innovation on Maternal Health (AIM) and are open access. Specifically, tools to guide SMM review panels are as follows:

- Severe Maternal Morbidity Review Form (+AIM) (California Department of Public Health, n.d.)

- Support After a Severe Maternal Event (+AIM) (American College of Obstetricians and Gynecologists, 2015)

Improving the data is a critical step in identifying evidence-based approaches in mending the maternal health safety net. Accurate and consistent data are essential to creating equity and a culture of safety.

STRENGTHENING COMMUNITY SERVICES

Collaboration in the Provision of Maternal Health Services

Community services to strengthen and mend the safety net need to be collaborative to achieve the best results. An example is collaboration between the Healthy Start program and Legal Aid organization. While Healthy Start seeks to protect the health of mothers and babies, legal aid services address the social determinants and environment in which mothers live, for example, housing, transportation, and access to community services and criminal justice counseling (Atkins, Heller, DeBartolo, & Sandel, 2014).

Primary Care Services

Primary care services also need to be located where women and their families live their lives. Federally qualified health centers (FQHCs) located in isolated or poorly serviced rural or urban areas are an essential part of community-based care (Smith, Johnson-Lawrence, Andrews, & Parker, 2017). Funds for FQHCs are allocated by the federal government to provide primary care in underserved areas.

One of the advantages of FQHCs is the involvement of the community, including a governing board that includes clients. The influence of this community-based board helps with the identification of services essential for a healthy community, such as the need for transportation to the center. Another advantage, affecting under- or uninsured women, is an income-based sliding scale fee for healthcare needs. The services at a FQHC offer access to a variety of providers, including nurses, advanced practice nurses, family practice and some specialty physicians, and public health professionals. FQHCs often integrate pharmacy, mental health, substance use, and oral health services in areas where economic, geographical, or cultural barriers limit access to affordable healthcare services. Often providers represent the cultural and ethnic groups of the community, increasing the potential for cultural competency and language fluency. In states with Medicaid expansion under the Patient Protection and Affordable Care Act (ACA), the majority of childbearing women are insured, as previously described in this book.

The expansion of Medicaid under the ACA allows FQHCs to serve 40% more patients than clinics in nonexpansion states. The higher operating revenues enable expansion of healthcare needed by postpartum women, such as behavioral/mental health and addiction services and oral healthcare. In states where FQHCs have adopted the ACA expansion, the quality of care has improved (Cole, Galárraga, Wilson, Wright, & Trivedi, 2017). The expanded Medicaid option under the ACA increases the role of the FQHC in both preconception and postpartum care.

Preconception Care

Preconception and interconception health issues can be addressed before pregnancy, decreasing the potential for preventable maternal mortality and SMM (Bello,

Rendon, & Arany, 2013; Carlin, Alfirevic, & Gyte, 2017; CDC, 2018). Examples of services provided include management of underlying cardiac conditions and hypertension, type 2 diabetes, mental health disorders, infections, HIV health maintenance, opioid and substance abuse, and intimate partner violence (IPV).

Postpartum Care

Medicaid expansion has had a positive impact in rural areas where growth in Medicaid coverage and decline in insurance coverage are greater than in urban areas. In states without ACA Medicaid expansion, both rural and urban areas have experienced declines in coverage (Kaiser Family Foundation, 2016, 2018).

Mental health issues, including opioid abuse, are prevalent in the postpartum period. Maternal mortality from mental health conditions is most likely to occur in the late postpartum period, accounting for 16.2% of all late pregnancy-related deaths occurring between 43 and 365 days (Building U.S. Capacity, 2018). Less than one in five addiction treatment centers specifically provide services for pregnant or postpartum women (Terplan, Longinaker, & Appel, 2015). This lack of treatment feeds into the cyclical pattern of incarceration (Sufrin, 2017). In states with Medicaid expansion, programs are in place that help mothers to combat opioid use with medication assisted therapy (MAT), behavioral health therapy, and mentor support. The need for continued innovations to provide safe and optimal care for mothers beyond the birth is part of the safety net.

Another concern is late-onset cardiomyopathy, especially among African American mothers (Howell et al., 2016; Irizarry et al., 2017). Ongoing fatigue may be more than just managing a newborn. Helping the HIV+ postpartum mother to keep her appointments and be well regulated with her medications is another challenge (Momplaisir, Storm, Nkwihoreze, Jayeola, & Jemmott, 2018). Screening and referring women in situations of IPV is a key initiative in expanded postpartum care. A critical public health problem, IPV is implicated in over 54% of childbearing-associated suicides and 45% of childbearing-associated homicides (Alhusen, Ray, Sharp, & Bullock, 2015; Wallace, Hoyert, Willams, & Mendola, 2016).

Postpartum Support Services

Perinatal home visitation programs are proposed as best practice for high-risk mothers, especially those in an environment of IPV. The Domestic Violence Enhanced Home Visitation Program (DOVE) was a multisite randomized control trial ($n = 239$) conducted from 2006 to 2012, evaluating home visitation among women experiencing perinatal IPV. It included screening and face-to-face, in-home brief counseling. The DOVE program was effective in reducing IPV among childbearing women in the intervention group at six points in time: 1, 3, 6, 12, 18, and 24 months postpartum ($p > 0.001$; Sharps et al., 2016).

Another service available in some areas to assist women with a successful transition to parenthood is the use of a certified postpartum doula. The presence of a doula beyond birth is a way to provide ongoing emotional support. Doulas can also provide help with breastfeeding and watch for signs of postpartum depression or other problems occurring in the late postpartum period.

Telehealth and Geocoding

Telehealth technology assists rural communities to gain access to care, especially for mothers without transportation. In some settings the cost of a telehealth visit is covered by Medicaid, reducing costs and emotional burden on the mother and her family. Privacy, convenience, and access to licensed and credentialed healthcare providers and therapists makes this innovative approach as effective as in-person services and counseling. The quality of care provided by telehealth is often equivalent to the services that would be rendered at distant locations, while reducing utilization of emergency room services for nonemergent conditions.

Geocoding is another innovative technological approach in mending the safety net. Using geographical information systems (GIS), communities can be mapped for risk, including maternal mortality, morbidity, and birth outcomes. The value of this mapping is the identification of communities that need to be targeted for enhanced services (Suplee, Bloch, Hillier, & Herbert, 2018).

In addition, having a real-time map of the community can identify those childbearing women who need extra support in coping with adverse neighborhood conditions and transportation challenges (Giurgescu et al., 2015).

The Safety Bundles for Postpartum Care

The Safety Bundles for Postpartum Care have been developed to help providers and institutions prevent maternal mortality and severe morbidity and offer management strategies. Vetted by the AIM, these open access tools, like the other safety bundles discussed previously in this book, provide consistency and best practices. The postpartum safety bundles are:

- Postpartum Care Basics for Maternal Safety: Transition From Maternity to Well-Woman Care (+AIM) (ACOG, 2018)

- Postpartum Care Basics for Maternal Safety: From Birth to the Comprehensive Postpartum Visit (+AIM) (ACOG, 2017).

These safety bundles help create equity and a safety net for childbearing women.

Freestanding Birth Centers

Freestanding birth centers (FSBCs) located in or very close to FQHCs are an emerging model, as demonstrated in the Strong Start Initiative (American Association of Birth Centers [AABC], 2018). Especially in underserved areas, this model can have an enhanced effect on creating a culture of equity and safety. Many women with Medicaid coverage, as well as private insurance, prefer birth center care. Outcomes are excellent for low-risk women (Alliman & Phillippi, 2016; Stapleton, Osborne, & Illuzzi, 2013). Positive outcomes among Medicaid beneficiaries in the Strong Start birth center sites, as described in Chapter 5, are particularly robust (AABC, 2018; Jolles et al., 2017). Most private insurances cover birth center facility and provider charges and hospital or physician practices that include birth center/midwifery-led care (AABC, 2015). In some states Medicaid coverage does not cover the costs (Edmonds, Mogul, & Shea, 2015). In states with enhanced Medicaid coverage with ACA, birth center care is more available.

The Developing Families Center, founded by Dr. Ruth Lubic, is located in a low-income neighborhood in Washington, DC. With many years of service to the community, this innovation center is the national model of an integrated nurse-midwife-managed primary healthcare/birth center (Lubic & Flynn, 2010). It has provided the foundation for national thinking about integration of community services. The model of the FQHC with an FSBC has been recommended as a viable safety net solution for low-risk women in isolated geographical areas and low-income urban settings (Wilkes & Alliman, 2017).

The next step, going forward, is to create a viable cost reimbursement system for birth centers. Going forward, AABC is proposing national legislation to create a federally funded demonstration project. The Birth Access Benefitting Improved Essential Facility Services (the BABIES Act) would provide birth center care in underserved areas with reimbursement comparable to the federal reimbursement model used by FQHCs (AABC, n.d.).

CHANGING THE PARADIGM IN SCHOOL-BASED HEALTH EDUCATION

Sex education is one of the most contentious aspects of school-based health education. Part of strengthening the safety net for childbearing is rethinking the concept of school-based health education. The delivery of "family life education" in grades K–12 is often overshadowed by the national debate on advocating for abstinence or teaching contraceptive methods. It is also customary to spend considerable educational energy on delivering messages about the usual culprits—illicit drugs, smoking, alcohol, and sexual activity. To reach American youth, a paradigm shift toward a self-directed life course model is needed. Other developed nations employ this approach in school-based health education with positive outcomes (Anderson, 2008).

Focus on Life Course Development

For many young persons, family life is not necessarily healthy or happy. The overarching themes in life course development need to be making individual choices and contributing to an equitable, just, and healthy society. Discussion of life choices needs to include all areas of life, not just sexuality. It needs to teach life skills for recognizing and managing socially destructive messages, like implicit bias, racism, gender discrimination, and fear of the "other." Including youth in designing this curriculum would give them voice. However, there are concerns about this approach. Some of these concerns are cost, time, and creating adversarial relationships among parents of different belief systems. Despite evidence to the contrary, public perception questions whether this approach would make a difference.

Health professionals, including nurses, doctors, health educators, and others, are powerful role models. They need to be physically present before students, giving correct information about health professional careers, counteracting the commonly incorrect information disseminated by school health fairs and counselors. One-on-one mentoring by health professionals, especially for those students most likely to be subject to racism, poverty, and discrimination, would help young persons in moving toward careers, including the health professions. An excellent example in the United States is the work of Shafia Monroe, executive director of International Center for Traditional Childbearing, located in Portland, Oregon. The project, Sistah Care, reaches out to primarily African American girls in middle school and high school with school-based education around career development, healthy living, and knowledge about healthy childbearing. The project includes practical experiences and community outreach by the young women (Shafia Monroe, personal communication, November 7, 2018).

A Life Course Journey

One day, I (BA) entered the public high school where I was the school nurse/health educator. I noticed one of my students, Susan, a sophomore who was 4 months pregnant, sitting in the hallway—her shoulders drooped and her head in her hands. The young persons in this school district had lived their lives in poverty, experiencing inequity and racism on a daily basis. A survival mechanism was a high index of suspicion. I tried to be very gentle with them, sensing their suspicions. Very softly I asked Susan if I could sit down beside her. She nodded her head. I asked her, "What's the matter, Susan?" She looked up, eyes full of pain, and said, "I want to die. I just want to die."

"Do you want to hurt yourself, Susan?" She nodded yes. "Have you thought about how you might do it?" She nodded no. My mind raced with all the protocols and instructions about threatened suicide and knowing, at this fragile moment, how easily trust could be shattered.

"I got some cookies in my office and I'm hungry. Want to have a cookie?" I asked her. She nodded yes. We finished the whole package and I wrote a vague permission slip for her missing two classes. That day I began a journey with one of the most beautiful persons I have ever known. She poured out her pain, her loneliness, her hopes for her baby, and her sense of despair. I did not initiate the rapid response suicide protocol. Rather, I met with her regularly, even as little as 2 minutes at times. We talked about her life, her life course to date, and what she wanted in her life. She wanted this baby, she wanted to live, and she wanted to finish school. One day she did not come to school and I was worried. Later that morning I learned that she had delivered a premature baby girl during the night. She was discharged from the hospital the next day while the baby remained in neonatal intensive care. I only saw Susan one time after that. A public health nurse followed her with home visits.

Four years later, in my new position as a nursing instructor at the local college, I was grading papers at my desk. Without knocking, a young woman entered my office with an adorable preschooler in tow. The woman announced, "I'm back." I looked at her, trying to remember her face.

"Don't you remember me? I'm Susan." Memories flooded me as I recalled the broken teenager who had munched on cookies with me.

"Susan, how wonderful to see you. Please have a seat." I winked at her and said, "I've got some cookies. Would you and your lovely little girl like some cookies?" She laughed and nodded yes as she sat down. Four-year-old Tina dived into the cookies.

Susan did not waste any words delivering her message: "Ever since I met you, I've wanted to be a nurse. So, I'm back. Will you teach me to be a nurse?" Four years later, with help from a scholarship, caring faculty, and peer mentors, as well as a lot of determination to set her life course, Susan graduated and passed the nursing board exam. She took a position as a staff nurse in a postpartum unit and eventually became the mother–baby nurse manager and a local leader in nursing. The last time I saw her she was a busy, active professional nurse raising a beautiful child.

SUMMARY

The public health safety net is very porous. At times, data are lost, services are inaccessible, and health education for American youth is tightly focused on sex education. The safety net fails to address preparation for a healthy life and future parenting. Mending the safety net for childbearing is one of the most important endeavors in meeting the *Healthy People 2020* goals. Supporting youth, mothers, and growing families is an essential part of creating a strong safety net necessary for a just and equitable society.

WHAT IF

This section poses critical questions and discussion points about the crippling of health and the loss of life among America's mothers. It is an opportunity to think creatively about how to mend the maternal health safety net using community-based strategies. Answers are deliberately not provided. The solutions to this national epidemic lie in interdisciplinary, imaginative conversation and problem solving. The authors invite the readers to consider these questions and add additional ones.

MENDING THE MATERNAL HEALTH SAFETY NET: COMMUNITY-BASED STRATEGIES

What is the relationship between the quality of maternal mortality and morbidity data and the public health safety net?

Identify key postpartum causes of mortality and morbidity.

Describe the timing of maternal mortality and morbidity in the postpartum.

Discuss the rationale for including 1st year postpartum mortality and morbidity data in the national database.

What are some specific ways to create equity in community-based services?

How could utilization of technology, like geocoding and telehealth, change equity in healthcare?

How do FQHCs and freestanding birth centers promote access to care?

Discuss life course theory as a model for changing the paradigm of school-based health education.

What can be done to strengthen and mend the public health safety net for childbearing women?

REFERENCES

Agrawal, P. (2015). Maternal mortality and morbidity in the United States of America. *Bulletin of the World Health Organization, 93*(3), 135. doi:10.2471/BLT.14.148627

Alhusen, J., Ray, E., Sharps, P., & Bullock, L. (2015). Intimate partner violence during pregnancy: Maternal and neonatal outcomes. *Journal of Women's Health, 24*(1), 100–106. doi:10.1089/jwh.2014.4872

Alliman, J., & Phillippi, J. (2016). Maternal outcomes in birth centers: An integrative review of the literature. *Journal of Midwifery and Women's Health, 61*(1), 21–51. doi:10.1111/jmwh.12356

American Association of Birth Centers. (n.d.). *BABIES Act: Birth access benefitting improved essential facility services* (pp. 1–3). Perkiomenville, PA: Author. Retrieved from https://c.ymcdn.com/sites/www.birthcenters.org/resource/resmgr/legislation_-_documents/BABIES_Act_Summary_-_4.27.18.pdf

American Association of Birth Centers. (2015). Update on AABC Medicaid survey of birth centers. *AABC News.* Retrieved from https://www.birthcenters.org/store/ViewProduct.aspx?ID=10046031

American Association of Birth Centers. (2018, November 9). *New government report recommends birth center care* [Press release]. Retrieved from https://www.birthcenters.org/news/426371/New-Government-Report-Recommends-Birth-Center-Care.htm

American College of Obstetricians and Gynecologists. (2015). Support after a severe maternal event (+AIM). Retrieved from https://safehealthcareforeverywoman.org/patient-safety-bundles/support-after-a-severe-maternal-event-supported-by-aim

American College of Obstetricians and Gynecologists. (2017). Postpartum care basics for maternal safety: From birth to the comprehensive postpartum visit (+AIM). Retrieved from https://safehealthcareforeverywoman.org/patient-safety-bundles/postpartum-care-basics-1

American College of Obstetricians and Gynecologists. (2018). Postpartum care basics for maternal safety: Transition from maternity to well-woman care (+AIM). Retrieved from https://safehealthcareforeverywoman.org/patient-safety-bundles/postpartum-care-basics-2

Anderson, B. (2008, May). *Assessment of midwifery practice and birth centers in Denmark, Iceland, Finland, Norway and Sweden.* Oral presentation to the Board of Directors. Perkiomenville, PA: American Association of Birth Center.

Atkins, D., Heller, S., DeBartolo, E., & Sandel, M. (2014). Medical-legal partnership and Healthy Start: Integrating civil legal aid services into public health advocacy. *Journal of Legal Medicine, 35*(1), 195–209. doi:10.1080/01947648.2014.885333

Bello, N., Rendon, I., & Arany, Z. (2013). The relationship between pre-eclampsia and peripartum cardiomyopathy: A systematic review and meta-analysis. *Journal of the American College of Cardiology, 62*(18), 1715–1723. doi:10.1016/j.jacc.2013.08.717

Bingham, D., Suplee, P., Morris, M., & McBride, M. (2018). Healthcare strategies for reducing pregnancy-related morbidity and mortality in the postpartum period. *The Journal of Perinatal and Neonatal Nursing, 32*(3), 241–249. doi:10.1097/JPN.0000 000000000344

Building U.S. Capacity to Review and Prevent Maternal Deaths. (2018). *Report from nine maternal mortality review committees.* Retrieved from http://reviewtoaction.org/Report from Nine MMRCs

California Department of Public Health. (n.d.). Severe maternal morbidity review (+AIM). Retrieved from https://safehealthcareforeverywoman.org/patient-safety-tools/severe-maternal-morbidity-review

Carlin, A., Alfirevic, Z., & Gyte, G. (2010). Interventions for treating peripartum cardiomyopathy to improve outcomes for women and babies. *Cochrane Database of Systematic Reviews,* (9). doi:10.1002/14651858.CD008589.pub2

Centers for Disease Control and Prevention. (2017a). Pregnancy mortality surveillance system. Retrieved from https://www.cdc.gov/reproductivehealth/maternalinfanthealth/pmss.html

Centers for Disease Control and Prevention. (2017b). Severe maternal morbidity in the United States. Retrieved from https://www.cdc.gov/reproductivehealth/maternalinfanthealth/severematernalmorbidity.html

Centers for Disease Control and Prevention. (2018). *HIV in the United States and dependent area.* Retrieved from https://www.cdc.gov/hiv/statistics/overview/ataglance.html

Chen, H.-Y., Chauhan, S., & Blackwell, S. (2018). Severe maternal morbidity and hospital cost among hospitalized deliveries in the United States. *American Journal of Perinatology, 35*(13), 1287–1296. doi:10.1055/s-0038-1649481

Cole, M., Galárraga, O., Wilson, I., Wright, B., & Trivedi, A. (2017). At federally funded health centers, Medicaid expansion was associated with improved quality of care. *Health Affairs, 36*(1), 40–48. doi:10.1377/hlthaff.2016.0804

Creanga, A., Berg, C., Ko, J., Farr, S., Tong, V., Bruce, F., & Callaghan, W. (2014). Maternal mortality and morbidity in the United States: Where are we now? *Journal of Women's Health, 23*(1), 3–9. doi:10.1089/jwh.2013.4617

Edmonds, B., Mogul, M., & Shea, J. (2015). Understanding low-income African American women's expectations, preferences, and priorities in prenatal care. *Family and Community Health, 38*(2), 149–157. doi:10.1097/FCH.0000000000000066

Giurgescu, C., Zenk, S., Templin, T., Engeland, C., Dancy, B., Park, C., . . . Misra, D. (2015). The impact of neighborhood environment, social support, and avoidance coping on depressive symptoms of pregnant African-American women. *Women's Health Issues, 25*(3), 294–302. doi:10.1016/j.whi.2015.02.001

Howell, E., Egorova, N., Balbierz, A., Zeitlin, J., & Hebert, P. (2016). Black-White differences in severe maternal morbidity and site of care. *American Journal of Obstetrics & Gynecology, 214*(1), 122.e1–122.e7. doi:10.1016/j.ajog.2015.08.019

Irizarry, O., Levine, L., Lewey, J., Boyer, T., Riis, V., Elovitz, M., & Arany, Z. (2017). Comparison of clinical characteristics and outcomes of peripartum cardiomyopathy between African American and non–African American women. *JAMA Cardiology, 2*(11), 1256–1260. doi:10.1001/jamacardio.2017.3574

Jolles, D., Langford, R., Stapleton, S., Cesario, S., Koci, A., & Alliman, J. (2017). Outcomes of childbearing Medicaid beneficiaries engaged in care at Strong Start birth center sites between 2012 and 2014. *Birth, 44*(4), 298–305. doi:10.1111/birt.12302

Kaiser Family Foundation. (2016). *State health facts: Health insurance coverage of the total population.* Retrieved from https://www.kff.org/other/state-indicator/total-population/?currentTimeframe=0&sortModel=%7B%22colId%22:%22Location%22,%22sort%22:%22asc%22%7D

Kaiser Family Foundation. (2018). *Where are states today? Medicaid and state eligibility levels for children, pregnant women, and adults.* Retrieved from https://www.kff.org/medicaid/fact-sheet/where-are-states-today-medicaid-and-chip

Lubic, R., & Flynn, C. (2010). The Family Health and Birth Center—A nurse–midwife-managed center in Washington, DC. *Alternative Therapies in Health and Medicine, 16*(5), 58–60.

MacDorman, M., Declercq, E., Cabral, H., & Morton, C. (2016). Recent increases in the U.S. maternal mortality rate: Disentangling trends from measurement issues. *Obstetrics & Gynecology, 128*, 447–455. doi:10.1097/AOG.0000000000001556

Momplaisir, F. M., Storm, D. S., Nkwihoreze, H., Jayeola, O., & Jemmott, J. B. (2018). Improving postpartum retention in care for women living with HIV in the United States. *AIDS, 32*(2), 133–142. doi:10.1097/QAD.0000000000001707

Sharps, P., Bullock, L., Campbell, J., Alhusen, J., Ghazarian, S., Bhandari, S., & Schminkey, D. (2016). Domestic violence enhanced perinatal home visits: The DOVE randomized clinical trial. *Journal of Women's Health, 25*(11), 1129–1138. doi:10.1089/jwh.2015.5547

Smith, L., Johnson-Lawrence, V., Andrews, M., & Parker, S. (2017). Opportunity for interprofessional collaborative care—Findings from a sample of federally qualified health center patients in the Midwest. *Public Health, 151,* 131–136. doi:10.1016/j.puhe.2017.07.009

St. Pierre, A., Zaharatos, J., Goodman, D., & Callaghan, W. (2018). Challenges and opportunities in identifying, reviewing, and preventing maternal deaths. *Obstetrics and Gynecology, 131*(1), 138–142. doi:10.1097/AOG.0000000000002417

Stapleton, S., Osborne, C., & Illuzzi, J. (2013). Outcomes of care in birth centers: Demonstration of a durable model. *Journal of Midwifery and Women's Health, 58*(1), 3–14. doi:10.1111/jmwh.12003

Sufrin, C. (2017). *Jailcare: Finding the safety net for women behind bars.* Oakland: University of California Press.

Suplee, P., Bloch, J., Hillier, A., & Herbert, T. (2018). Using geographic information systems to visualize relationships between perinatal outcomes and neighborhood characteristics when planning community interventions. *Journal of Obstetric, Gynecologic & Neonatal Nursing, 47*(2), 158–172. doi:10.1016/j.jogn.2018.01.002

Terplan, M., Longinaker, N., & Appel, L. (2015). Women-centered drug treatment services and need in the United States, 2002–2009. *American Journal of Public Health, 105*(11), e50–e54. doi:10.2105/AJPH.2015.302821

Ungar, L. (2018, September 20). What states aren't doing to save new mothers' lives. *USA Today.* Retrieved from https://www.usatoday.com/in-depth/news/investigations/deadly-deliveries/2018/09/19/maternal-death-rate-state-medical-deadly-deliveries/547050002

Wallace, M., Hoyert, D., Williams, C., & Mendola, P. (2016). Pregnancy-associated homicide and suicide in 37 US states with enhanced pregnancy surveillance. *American Journal of Obstetrics and Gynecology, 215*(3), 364.e1–364.e10. doi:10.1016/j.ajog.2016.03.040

Wilkes, A., & Alliman, J. (2017). Enhanced care services and health homes. In L. Cole & M. Avery (Eds.), *Freestanding birth centers: Innovation, evidence, optimal outcomes* (pp. 229–247). New York, NY: Springer Publishing Company.

World Health Organization, United Nations International Children's Emergency Fund, United Nations Population Fund, World Bank Group, & United Nations Population Division. (2015). *Trends in maternal mortality: 1990 to 2015: Estimates by WHO, UNICEF, UNFPA, World Bank Group and the United Nations Population Division.* Geneva, Switzerland: World Health Organization. Retrieved from http://www.who.int/reproductivehealth/publications/monitoring/maternal-mortality-2015/en

A ROAD MAP FOR NURSING ADVOCACY AND PRACTICE

BARBARA A. ANDERSON | LISA R. ROBERTS

OBJECTIVES

At the end of this chapter, the reader will be able to:

1. Summarize factors influencing maternal health, morbidity, and mortality in the United States.

2. Examine themes in the key informant interviews.

3. Describe a road map for nursing advocacy and practice that promotes maternal health in the United States.

MATERNAL MORTALITY AND MORBIDITY: CONTRIBUTING FACTORS

This book has sought to examine factors contributing to the high maternal mortality and morbidity in the United States in light of nursing implications for advocacy and practice. In conversation with many persons about this work, we have been asked to provide the answer to this question: What is the reason why the United States is experiencing this crisis in maternal health? The only viable answer is: It's complicated. There is no one reason or quick solution. It is an entrenched, multifaceted issue touching on many realms of life in America. This final chapter summarizes some of the contributing factors.

The Poor Health of the People

As described throughout this book, the general health of Americans is poor. Longevity is shorter, compared to other developed nations (Woolf & Aron, 2013). American mothers are no exception to this national profile. The rise in maternal mortality, severe morbidity, and near miss events have been well documented (Amnesty International, 2011; Centers for Disease Control and

Prevention [CDC], 2017a, 2017b; Global Burden of Disease Study Maternal Mortality Collaborators, 2016). The United States now has the highest maternal mortality of any developed nation (Central Intelligence Agency, 2018). Causes of maternal mortality and morbidity have shifted. American mothers, reflecting the health of the nation, increasingly have chronic diseases and comorbidities (Creanga, 2018).

A Divided Society

The nation is divided along many lines. Social and economic variables undermine access and equity in healthcare. Early life course has implications for individual health throughout life (Halfon, Larson, Lu, Tullis, & Russ, 2014). Over half of all births in the United States are financed by Medicaid, pointing to the high level of poverty and limited income across a wide swatch of American mothers (Smith et al., 2017). Racism, implicit bias, and lack of national consensus on healthcare access for all persons influence equity in healthcare. The *Healthy People 2020* national agenda focuses on the critical issue of healthcare equity (see www.cdc.gov/dhdsp/hp2020.htm).

Gaps in Healthcare and Public Health Services

The United States has no national health system. Privatized systems restrict access to care. The public health system is highly subject to legislative whims. Government-administered services, that is, Medicare/Medicaid, are often in competition with the privatized system. Coverage gaps exist, putting many women at risk due to lack of access to care. The Patient Protection and Affordable Care Act (ACA) has expanded services for Medicaid in those states that have adopted this legislation (ACA, 2010).

A growing shortage of maternal healthcare providers, the lack of diversification of the workforce that reflects the face of America, and closure of rural facilities continue to be a problem (Dawley & Walsh, 2016; Kozhimannil et al., 2015). Scaling up the availability of midwifery care, especially in rural and underserved areas, is a widely proposed solution (Homer et al., 2014; Kennedy et al., 2018).

The culture of safety for maternal care revolves around high levels of technological intervention rather than promotion of the safer option, physiologic birth. Many health professionals have never seen or participated in a completely physiologic birth. The lack of uptake of the maternal patient safety bundles (40% of hospitals) and lack of consistency in managing obstetrical emergencies point to the need for continued education of all maternal healthcare providers (California Maternal Quality Care Collaborative [CMQCC], 2018; CBS News, 2018; Council on Patient Safety in Women's Health Care, 2018). Positive birth outcomes among Medicaid beneficiaries in the Strong Start initiative are particularly robust in promoting physiologic birth (American Association of Birth Centers [AABC], 2018).

Maternal Health Statistics: Inadequate Data

Lack of consistent and analogous data prevent comparison of public health, health-care, and patient outcomes from state to state, or with other nations (Agrawal, 2015; MacDorman & Declercq, 2018; Woolf & Aron, 2013). While infant health, mortality, and adverse outcomes are generally well recorded, reporting of maternal health statistics are often inconsistent. Data are managed by individual states often with different criteria. Only about 50% of the states have maternal review boards (Clark & Belfort, 2017). Standardized and shared data using common terminology as well as state and local maternity review boards could become the most efficient means of obtaining data (St. Pierre, Zaharatos, Goodman, & Callaghan, 2018). A national maternal health review board is recommended (Clark & Belfort, 2017). The CDC has taken leadership in development and training for maternal mortality review (Building U.S. Capacity to Review and Prevent Maternal Deaths, 2018). Severe maternal morbidity (SMM) is much more prevalent than maternal mortality. Systematic data collection on maternal morbidity is also lacking (Agrawal, 2015; Creanga et al., 2014). The Council on Patient Safety in Women's Health Care (2018) disseminates tools to guide SMM institutional review panels.

Motherhood in America: The Social Environment

The current antinatalist social environment has been discussed in both popular media and professional publications, as the birth rate declines. In May 2018, the *Huffington Post* published a thoughtful piece entitled "Everyone is missing a key reason the U.S. birth rate is declining" (Peck, 2018). The author described the unsupportive social climate for raising a family in America. As noted in the preface to this book, mothers in America continue to be defined in terms of the "other" as *vessel* for child health, *cause* for preterm and ill babies, and *subcategory* of women's healthcare. These social presentations of the mantle of motherhood impact policy and practices across many domains of American life, presenting risks to maternal health and life.

Family Leave

Family-friendly policies are common in most developed nations. The United States does not have a universal, enforceable family leave policy. Employers are at will to grant leave or not. With many families struggling economically, mothers often return to full-time work well before adjusting to parenthood and recovering vital energy. Extended family may not be in the immediate region to help with infant care and manage the household. Fathers may have limited or no time off work or may not be able to take any loss of pay with a growing family. Affordable and reliable child care is an enormous issue and expense.

Currently there is an increasing trend toward a high level of mortality and morbidity in the 1st year postpartum. The CDC seeks to capture the data on pregnancy-related mortality, which encompasses not only pregnancy and birth but a full year postpartum. For example, pregnancy-related cardiomyopathy, especially among African American mothers, often has an initial onset in the extended postpartum period. The postpartum is now the new frontier for research in maternal health.

Employment Climate

In the work environment, there may be limited tolerance for the needs of new parents. Although many work settings provide family leave, sick leave to care for ill children, and private areas to breastfeed or to pump and store breast milk, not all companies are so generous. In one employment setting, I (BA) proposed using a small room, storing old files and other paraphernalia, as a breastfeeding/pumping room for a number of new mothers in the organization. I explained the growing trend for baby-friendly hospitals, workplaces, and restaurants. The first person on the facilities committee responded, "Why don't they just go to the bathroom and sit on the toilet to pump?" Another said, "They will just use that space to take longer breaks." A third person questioned why we were even having this conversation, noting that new mothers were pretty useless as employees.

Fortunately, public advocacy by professionals, parents, and citizen groups and some high-profile legal cases are creating change. We did get the breastfeeding space, complete with a donated rocking chair, changing table, a small refrigerator for milk storage, and some lovely pieces of art to hang on the wall. Nothing happened, however, until I offered to come in on my day off to clean out the room, buy the paint, and paint the walls. It took one day to clean, paint, move in donated items, and decorate the room as many employees volunteered to help, including one of the members of the facilities committee!

Social Messages About Childbearing

Social messages about childbearing abound in every culture. Sometimes these messages are about the mystery of birth and the value of the mother. An Islamic proverb states, "Paradise is beneath the feet of mothers" (Prophet Muhammad as cited in Mischler, 2017). Sometimes the social messages are not so positive. Both authors recall being called "cute," as strangers patted our pregnant bellies—maybe a vocabulary deficiency or perhaps patronizing. "Don't worry, you will soon get your figure back," said one person, no doubt not realizing that pregnancy also creates a body shape that is beautiful.

Condescending messages also target the mind and the emotions. "You are just emotional because you are pregnant" is a common piece of advice, as if life stresses, for example, financial woes or relationship stresses, can be explained so simply. Messages about the intensity of pain are rife, "This will be the worst pain you've ever experienced. I thought I was going to die." Offhanded or "dumbing down" messages are sometimes delivered by health professionals, assuming limited intelligence or knowledge. Explaining the complexities of childbearing in a respectful, non-judgmental manner is one of the most important factors in the provider–mother dyad. The media propagates the image of hysterical maternal response to birth, as witnessed by the manner in which childbirth is often portrayed. The scenario is a pregnant woman in excruciating pain as her hapless partner drives frantically to the hospital. They enter the emergency room where someone, usually an older male physician, "rescues" her by "delivering" her baby. The couple then is engrossed in admiration for the person who caught the baby and name the child after this hero. The delivery of the placenta does not make it into the script.

Social media messaging can also be very positive. Many smartphone apps, You-Tube videos, and films seek to promote health-affirming, culturally contextualized messages for American mothers. Usually these messages are respectful and infor-mative. This kind of social media is critically needed and often one of the best ways that maternal health providers can reach childbearing women. Some key organiz-ations that support this approach are the American Academy of Nursing (AAN), the American College of Nurse-Midwives (ACNM), the American College of Ob-stetricians and Gynecologists (ACOG), and the Association of Women's Health, Obstetric and Neonatal Nurses (AWHONN; Amankwaa et al., 2018; see Appendix A for additional resources).

A ROAD MAP: NURSING IMPLICATIONS FOR ADVOCACY AND PRACTICE

The Foundations of Equity in Maternal Care

Nobel Peace Prize Laureate and former secretary-general of the United Nations Kofi Annan made the memorable statement, "When women thrive, all of society bene-fits, and succeeding generations are given a better start in life" ("Commemorating Women's Day," 2003, para. 1). When mothers fail to thrive, or even survive, no one benefits. It is estimated that an end to preventable maternal deaths could be achieved by 2035 in nearly all nations if strategically integrated actions are adopted (Bergevin, Faveau, & McKinnon, 2015). In the United States, one action helping women to thrive is the ACA, a social disrupter that has opened dialogue and debate about healthcare, including that offered to mothers. Medicaid expansion has furthered access to mater-nal care. Freestanding birth centers are now recommended by the federal government as a key way of facilitating physiologic birth for women at low risk. Initiatives under-taken by the CMQCC have proven effective in significantly reducing maternal mor-tality in California and in stimulating development of safety bundles across the nation.

The nursing profession is central to implementing the road map toward equity. As the largest cadre of health professionals in the nation, nurses provide a substan-tial amount of care to America's mothers. However, the current nursing shortage, at all levels in the United States, threatens the availability of maternal healthcare as well as the stability of the American healthcare system (American Association of

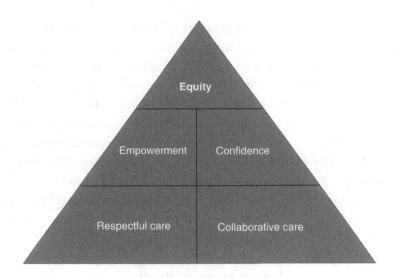

FIGURE 9.1 Foundations of equity in maternal care.

Colleges of Nursing [AACN], 2010). The 2010 call to action, *The Future of Nursing: Leading Change, Advancing Health* asks for the full utilization of knowledge and skills possessed by American nurses, including those with advanced practice skills (Institute of Medicine and Robert Wood Johnson Foundation, 2010). The AACN calls for national action on the nursing workforce issues, stagnated with inadequate numbers of applicants admitted to nursing educational programs (AACN, 2010). Implementing the road map to healthcare equity depends upon adequate numbers of healthcare providers, including nurses.

The U.S. healthcare system continues to place maternal health on the periphery (Halfon et al., 2014). Cultural and systemic change must occur before mothers in America can thrive and the *Healthy People 2020* goal of healthcare equity can be reached. We propose four foundational strategies toward reaching this goal:

- Respectful healthcare
- Collaborative teamwork
- Empowering and educating mothers
- Building maternal confidence in the childbearing process (see Figure 9.1.)

These strategies can foster a healthcare environment that builds healthcare equity and where mothers can thrive.

Implementing the Road Map Toward Equitable Healthcare

In examining each of these strategies, we conducted key informant interviews among maternal healthcare providers. We interviewed practitioners in different professional roles in order to obtain varying perspectives and to reinforce the essential principle of collaboration among maternal healthcare providers. Each interview exemplifies one of the four strategies and reflects upon implications for nursing advocacy and practice.

Respectful Care

Reproductive coercion, negating maternal autonomy in decision making, is a violation of the human rights of childbearing women and a kind of gender-based violence (ACOG, 2013; Fay & Yee, 2018). The 2010 landmark report *Exploring Evidence for Disrespect and Abuse in Facility-Based Childbirth* examined disrespect and abuse of childbearing women in maternity care systems across the world (Bowser & Hill, 2010). This key document explored human rights violations suffered by childbearing women, ranging from systemic and provider services to policy, law, and government. This document was formative in the development of the White Ribbon Alliance charter entitled *Respectful Maternity Care: The Universal Rights of Childbearing Women*. This global charter identifies seven categories of disrespect and abuse with corresponding rights of childbearing women:

- Physical abuse—Freedom from harm and ill treatment
- Nonconsented care—Information, informed consent, refusal, choices, companionship
- Nonconfidential care—Confidentiality, privacy
- Nondignified care and verbal abuse—Dignity, respect
- Discrimination—Equality, freedom from discrimination, equitable care
- Abandonment or denial of care—Timely care
- Detention in facilities—Liberty, autonomy, self-determination, freedom from coercion (White Ribbon Alliance, 2012)

Respectful care is a foundational strategy in promoting equity in maternal healthcare. This was the theme that emerged from the first key informant interview (see Key Informant Interview 9.1).

KEY INFORMANT INTERVIEW 9.1

RESPECTFUL CARE

DR. JOAN MACEACHEN, MD, MPH

Introduction of the Informant

Dr. Joan MacEachen is a family practice physician providing obstetrical care in rural Alaska. Joan is employed by a Native Alaskan tribal health clinic providing on-site and village outreach services to Alaska Natives and other populations in the community as needed.

(continued)

(continued)

Other populations served are military families, Alaskan settlers, Filipinos working in the local fish cannery, and those without health insurance. Much of Joan's work is done with Alaska Natives, a population who has historically experienced significant racism and inequity at the hands of the dominant White population. Joan has many years of providing maternal healthcare to Native American/Alaska Native women around the nation.

Description of the Population Served

Joan manages the care of many mothers with obesity, hypertension, gestational diabetes, and preeclampsia. She sees many women using marijuana and alcohol during pregnancy and a few using cocaine and methamphetamines. The drugs are smuggled to outlying villages via the daily airplane supply lines. Tribal funding of healthcare assures that Native Alaska mothers have accessibility to primary care. Preconception, prenatal, and postnatal care is offered through rotating provider visits to the villages with on-site community health aides (CHAs) monitoring general health. Joan attends births at the centralized site, a Level 1 hospital. Low-risk women and, as much as possible, high-risk women with comorbidities come to the centralized site 1 month in advance of the expected date of delivery to await the birth. Cesarean section at this site is low, even among those women with comorbidities.

Evidence of Respectful Care

Joan described the concern of the mothers in leaving their villages 1 month prior to giving birth as many have young children left behind with relatives or friends. This pattern interferes with maternal nurturance, the protection of children from potential sexual abuse, and sharing the birth experience with the baby's father. Nonetheless, mothers choose to come the centralized site to give birth as they have a long-standing, respectful relationship with Joan. She describes her approach to care as follows: "I try to be very gentle in advising a mother about the effects of drugs and alcohol not only on the baby but also on her health." She also stated, "It is very important to respect her choices about her birth and listen to her worries about leaving young children behind. I wish we could offer community birth, but we don't have the facilities or personnel in these very remote villages. We are fortunate to have the CHAs keeping an eye on the health of the community."

I have been side-by-side with Joan in a number of situations around the world, including rural Alaskan villages. She exemplifies cultural humility and deep respect of those with whom she works and provides care. She models respectful care in practice.

Interview by Barbara Anderson, September 21, 2018

Collaborative Teamwork

High-performing teams that work collaboratively improve health outcomes for mothers (Mitchell et al., 2012; Task Force on Collaborative Practice, 2016). While midwives alone can achieve remarkable maternal mortality reductions, the collaborative care model provided by midwives and obstetricians increases the impact (Bartlett, Weissman, Gubin, Patton-Molitors, & Friberg, 2014; Waldman, Kennedy, & Kendig, 2012). A high-performing, collaborative care team is characterized by:

- Mutual respect and trust among team members
- Nonhierarchic communication
- Valuing each team member's skills
- Sharing responsibility in decision making (Mitchell et al., 2012)

Best practices with a collaborative care model include the capacity to learn from one another, recognize disagreement, and value differences in thinking processes and approaches (Shekelle et al., 2013; Hutchison et al., 2011; Kennedy & Waldman, 2012). The collaborative care model is one of the strongest approaches in addressing the social determinants contributing to maternal mortality and morbidity and in promoting healthcare equity. Collaborative care was the theme that was described in the second key informant interview (see Key Informant Interview 9.2).

KEY INFORMANT INTERVIEW 9.2

COLLABORATIVE CARE

DR. JESSICA ILLUZZI, MD, MS, FACOG

Introduction of the Informant

Dr. Jessica Illuzzi is an obstetrician-gynecologist on faculty at Yale-New Haven School of Medicine. She is the section chief of the obstetric/midwifery section and medical director of the Vidone Birthing Center, St. Raphael Campus, Yale-New Haven Hospital, a collaborative faculty practice of obstetricians and certified nurse-midwives. She is on the board of directors of the American Association of Birth Centers.

Description of the Population Served

In collaboration with nurse-midwives and labor-delivery nurses, Jessica manages the care of low- and high-risk mothers from varied populations. This site is a training center for medical and midwifery students. A doula program, including volunteer doulas for women who cannot pay, provides additional support. The population served includes 70% Medicaid funded and 30% private pay. All mothers in this service receive midwifery care. The focus is physiologic birth, striving for delayed labor admission until 6 cm (active labor); low use of epidural anesthesia; use of nitrous oxide; full inclusion of the family even with complications; doula support for normal and complicated births; liberal fluids; active movement during labor; intermittent auscultation, unless otherwise contraindicated; and no separation of the baby from parents, including skin-to-skin care after the birth.

(continued)

(continued)

The cesarean rate is low, more so among Blacks and Latina mothers than White mothers. To avoid placental issues (i.e., accreta) among mothers with prior cesarean birth, the vaginal birth after cesarean (VBAC) rate is high. External cephalic version is attempted with breech, with obstetricians gaining skill in this procedure to facilitate cephalic birth. The service provides high-risk care to women with comorbidities and complications. Common problems are obesity, hypertension, gestational diabetes, preeclampsia, depression, substance abuse, intimate partner violence (IPV), unstable housing, and homelessness.

Evidence of Collaborative Care

Jessica stated, "The model of care is collaborative, nonhierarchical, choice centered, and physiologic. Emergency care is available with an obstetrician, midwife, and surgical team always in house. Every mother has a midwife. The mother is the center of the team that makes joint decisions on care. One team member is designated as family communicator." Jessica described that the team member with the highest skill in a situation manages the care. For instance, the team leader for a shoulder dystocia may be the certified nurse-midwife (CNM) or it could be the charge nurse managing the logistics of a crash cesarean. The social worker may lead the team when a woman is experiencing IPV. The mother is offered shelter in the birthing center until community services are arranged. The team carefully watches postpartum mothers due to awareness of the growing trend of high postpartum mortality and morbidity from cardiomyopathy. Jessica describes this model of care as promoting high functioning among the team, but most importantly, "A midwife, a nurse, and a doctor for every mother."

Interview by Barbara Anderson, October 22, 2018

Empowerment

Living in an environment that denigrates an individual or a population group takes its toll, creating chronic stress (Cheng & Solomon, 2014). Some maternal healthcare providers contribute to this stress by making assumptions about lack of competence, particularly related to race or culture (Williams, 2016). This assumption is palpable, creating inequity and eroding trust. Conversely, equity is supported when healthcare providers encourage a sense of empowerment. Dr. Dora Barilla, DrPH, CHES, president and cofounder of the California community-based organization HC2 Strategies described building empowerment, "We need to make sure that our care is appropriate for the individual and the culture that we're serving and that we are helping people to build skills in navigating the health care system" (Personal communication, October 10, 2018).

Empowerment is also built by community networks that recognize the mother's need to be cared for in her transition to motherhood. Dr. Barilla told this powerful story:

An Iraqi immigrant mother who had just given birth made a comment I will never forget. The mother told me that in Iraq, the community never leaves a mother alone after a baby is born, because "that's when the evil comes." This is such a wise cultural tradition. (Personal communication, October 10, 2018)

Empowerment comes from within, it cannot be bestowed on another, but it can be fostered and encouraged. It begins with respect. When a mother's questions and concerns are negated or pushed aside, the messages projected are "dumbing down" or "inability to know one's own needs." This negation can occur overtly or with the subtlest of nonverbal cues. On the other hand, acknowledging the validity of questions and concerns promotes the mother's sense of empowerment. Listening to her wisdom and encouraging her to make her own best decisions create genuine and equitable communication. Even if the mother lacks a sense of confidence and empowerment, she can learn these health-promoting skills in the presence of a healthcare provider who believes in her. Healthcare providers who seek to empower are promoting healthcare equity. Empowerment was the theme that arose in the third key informant interview (see Key Informant Interview 9.3).

KEY INFORMANT INTERVIEW 9.3

EMPOWERMENT

SHAFIA MONROE, DEM, MPH, CDT

Introduction of the Informant

Shafia Monroe is president of Shafia Monroe Consulting-Birthing CHANGE, located in Portland, Oregon. She is a public health professional, midwife, doula trainer, cultural competency trainer, author, and public speaker. Her leadership and advocacy for birth justice have resulted in numerous changes in birth practices. A *sagefemme*, midwife, and wise woman.

Description of the Population Served

Shafia serves many populations. The theme of empowerment threads through her work. Full Circle Doula Training teaches skills in labor and postpartum doula care, focusing on the doula as a presence in the life of the community. Her advocacy efforts were pivotal to legislation for doula funding for Medicaid-funded mothers in the state of Oregon. She founded the Sistah Care project, described in Chapter 8, guiding adolescent, primarily Black girls, to build confidence and empowerment. Some of these young women are now doulas and midwives, but even more importantly, she helped them to find their voices as mothers. She has promoted physiologic birth, helping mothers to feel empowered, normal, and competent in listening to their own wisdom.

(continued)

(continued)

Evidence of Empowerment

In a nation that does not have a robust safety net for childbearing women, Shafia gave examples of how women learn the words of empowerment. This begins with health education to understand the normalcy of childbearing and awareness of danger signs. Built upon this knowledge are skills in asking questions, insisting on being listened to, overcoming passivity, and advocating for self. She described a young, hypertensive Black woman who understood her risk for preeclampsia and potential cardiomyopathy. She began to experience headaches, ankle swelling, and shortness of breath. Her healthcare provider told her these were just the discomforts of pregnancy. She returned home but the symptoms persisted. Making a decision to take charge of her health and her life, she returned to the clinic. She asked pointed questions about her condition and insisted on being heard. She stated, "I do not feel right (normal) and I want to live to raise my child!" Her words had a powerful effect on the healthcare provider who further investigated her symptoms, resulting in immediate action to avert a disastrous outcome. How different from the life course story of Tony in Chapter 2, who tried to advocate for herself, was not listened to, and ended up with permanent cardiac damage and cardiomyopathy. Shafia ended the interview by saying, "I teach them to speak truth to power." How could I keep from singing when I heard her use this term of empowerment so foundational for healthcare equity?

Interview by Barbara Anderson, November 7, 2018

Building Maternal Confidence

To build a mother's confidence for physiologic birth, healthcare providers must recognize that women's bodies are designed to do just that. It is essential to move away from a risk-based model, that is, intervention as the safest route for every mother, and adopt physiologic birth as normative. This philosophical stance is critical to decreasing the high frequency of primary cesarean birth (Neerland, 2018).

The confidence of health providers in the physiologic process is palpable to mothers and influences their confidence. In addition to trusting their healthcare providers, mothers build confidence in their innate ability to give birth by education, social support, and a safe, comfortable environment (Neerland, 2018). Mothers with confidence for physiologic birth are better prepared to engage as partners in decision making, an important step in empowerment. The physiologic model as normative, backed by a safety net as needed, provides a base for improving maternal mortality and morbidity (Neerland, 2018). Maternal health nurses are key health professionals in leading this cultural shift. At the bedside, they are in touch with the mother's needs and can advocate for the mother to members of the team. They are in a pivotal position to advocate for patience in the birthing process. They also highly influence the mother's confidence. Nurses who inspire confidence in physiologic birth provide a base for building equity in maternal healthcare. Building maternal confidence was the theme identified in the fourth key informant interview (see Key Informant Interview 9.4).

KEY INFORMANT INTERVIEW 9.4

BUILDING MATERNAL CONFIDENCE

JULIA DE SOUZA, BSN, RN

Introduction of the Informant

Julia De Souza, Intrapartum Clinical Nursing Faculty, is an experienced labor and delivery nurse and clinical nursing instructor practicing in a Level 1 hospital, part of a regional referral center for high-risk pregnancies.

Description of the Population Served

Julia cares for laboring mothers in a high-intervention setting with a "better safe than sorry" stance. The maternity care team is composed of physicians, nurses, and medical residents. It is a teaching site for medical and nursing students. Julia stated, "We do have some doula patients but not frequently because our mothers are increasingly unhealthy or high risk. There aren't many that don't have some kind of history that can make their pregnancy high risk or dangerous." This setting is not optimal for low-risk women desiring physiologic birth. Julia continued, "We do allow the mother to tell us what she desires for her birth experience. Unless it's contraindicated by some kind of high-risk issue, there's no reason not to do it." Julia understands that physiologic birth is the safer option if possible. At a teaching hospital, maternal health nurses may have a substantial role in advocating for care and find their suggestions better received than in other settings. Julia reflected, "The residents rely on the nurses, but as they progress, there is more pushback. Our attending physicians, for the most part, are respectful of our advocacy."

Evidence of Building Maternal Confidence

Julia described the admission process as an opportunity for the nurse to assess a woman's desire, knowledge, and confidence for physiologic birth. She constantly assesses and educates mothers in labor about their progress, empowering them to make choices about their care. She described one mother who had been pushing for a long time and the physician was suggesting a cesarean. The mother did not want to have a cesarean. The baby's heart rate was fine and the mother wanted to keep trying. Julia advocated to the physician, who replied, "Okay, she can keep trying until we absolutely think it's best to do the C-section." Julia used all her skills to avoid the fear–tension–pain cycle that could interrupt the physiologic process. She directed the mother to "Focus on my voice; look at my face" when she had hard contractions, instilling confidence and helping her to stay calm. She used comfort measures to ease her pain and encouraged the family to surround the mother with their comforting presence. In a high-intervention culture, Julia is a change agent for building confidence in physiologic birth.

Interview by Lisa Roberts, November 15, 2018

Equity

Healthcare providers are significant role models for embracing and modeling a culture of justice and healthcare equity. We have proposed four strategies toward reaching the goal of healthcare equity:

- Respectful healthcare
- Collaborative teamwork
- Empowering and educating mothers
- Building maternal confidence in the childbearing process

We have presented interviews with key informants describing their important efforts toward healthcare equity. Each interview contained rich, detailed data, incorporating all of the strategies and characterized by equity. In reviewing the themes that emerged in each interview, we focused on one strategy per interview. This approach allowed for in-depth focus on each strategy. In the final key informant interview, we integrate all the strategies as an exemplar of a healthcare environment characterized by equity. The inequitable death and sickness of American mothers is embedded in the social determinants of health, especially racism. Changing the paradigm to one of equity requires attention to these social determinants and consciously implementing all the strategies for healthcare equity (see Key Informant Interview 9.5).

KEY INFORMANT INTERVIEW 9.5

EQUITY

DR. LAKIETA EDWARDS, DNP, RN, CNM, WHNP-BC

Introduction of the Informant

Dr. Lakieta Edwards is the first Black certified nurse-midwife to provide care in a freestanding birth center in Illinois. She practices full-scope midwifery in hospital and birth center settings.

Description of the Population Served

Dr. Edwards serves a predominately Hispanic (57%) and Black (39%) low-income population. Among the Hispanic population, about 30% do not have legal status and there are also DACA (Dreamers) among her clientele. Lakieta is fluent in both English and Spanish. Unstable housing, "invisible homelessness," that is, transitory living with others or in shelters, job insecurity, and homelessness are common. Intimate partner violence (IPV), history of incarceration, incarcerated partners, history of childhood sexual abuse, unsafe neighborhoods, stray bullets, and fear of violence from law enforcement are issues. Comorbidities include obesity, prepregnancy hypertension, preeclampsia, preexisting

(continued)

(*continued*)

cardiomyopathy, diabetes, gestational diabetes, anemia with poor diet and food insecurity, depression, and substance abuse. Lakieta stated, "Unremitting stress is baseline and it does not take much to snap." She described racism and gaps in service as the greatest contributors to inequity and stated that the input of mothers needs to be included in finding solutions to the maternal health crisis.

Evidence of Equity

Midwifery-centered birth center care or collaborative care in hospitals can help to provide respectful care and confidence in physiologic birth. Promoting the mother's best efforts in physiologic birth, regardless of her comorbidities, contributes to the mother's sense of empowerment and safety. A sense of safety is often greater in the birth center, as many mothers have vivid, recurring trauma and posttraumatic stress disorder after witnessing the death of loved ones in hospitals, frequently due to gang violence. Lakieta described the need for trauma-informed care among healthcare providers who complain about noncompliance but do not ask why it is occurring. She stated, "The mothers are trying and sometimes the healthcare providers and the hospital put barriers in their way." She described a bleeding pregnant woman who brought her 2-year-old with her to the hospital. She was reprimanded for doing so. She responded that she was a responsible mother and could not leave her 2-year-old alone. She spoke up and advocated for herself. Sometimes mothers just do not have childcare or transportation. Lakieta described the critical importance of mothers connecting with their providers for consistent care, especially with the high risk for cardiac and sepsis complications in the postpartum. She also discussed the need for mothers to connect culturally with the provider and emphasized the need for more Black and Hispanic midwives. All the strategies for equity—respectful care, collaborative care, empowerment, and confidence—are present. Lakieta is a midwife who embraces and is a role model for health equity.

Interview by Barbara Anderson, September 26, 2018

SUMMARY

The level of maternal mortality and SMM in the United States is at unconscionably high levels. In a nation of unparalleled wealth, the issues of inadequate data, a difficult social environment for childbearing and childrearing, the healthcare provider workforce shortage, and the social determinants that undermine health need to be examined from the perspectives of justice and equity. The traditional pattern of maternal healthcare frequently does not consider the disruption and danger of undermining social determinants, especially the deadly effect of racism. Focus on the social determinants of health is essential. Early life experiences, social, psychological, and environmental factors are critical social determinants. Examining these factors from a life course theory perspective can help healthcare providers understand the gestalt of women's lives.

Supporting political will, advocating for justice, and striving for healthcare equity are the responsibility and the privilege of those who wear the mantle of healthcare provider. As stated by Midwife Lakieta Edwards, "With the key stakeholders: women, their families, public health, nurses, midwives, doctors, birth workers, government officials, and the community, we can turn these outcomes around" (Personal communication, December 4, 2018). Nurses, as the largest cadre of health professionals, are consistently rated as the most trusted professionals in the nation. The implications for maternal health advocacy and utilization of best practices are clear. We are trusted, we are skilled, the time is now, and, in collaboration with our healthcare colleagues, we must do it.

WHAT IF

This section poses critical questions about the maternal health crisis in America discussed throughout this book. It is an opportunity to think innovatively about solutions posed and incubate new solutions. The information drawn together here provides a foundation for interdisciplinary, imaginative conversation and problem solving. The authors invite the readers to consider these questions and add additional ones.

A ROAD MAP FOR NURSING ADVOCACY AND PRACTICE

Is it possible to separate practice and advocacy? Why or why not?

How do the factors that contribute to the nursing workforce shortage and distribution impact the stability of the healthcare system in the United States?

How can advocacy change the team composition of maternal healthcare team?

What has been the impact of replication of the CMQCC across the nation?

What are some ways that community and professional organizations can hold government and healthcare providers accountable for quality and availability of maternal health services?

Discuss the model Foundations for Equity in Maternal Care from a cultural shift perspective.

REFERENCES

Agrawal, P. (2015). Maternal mortality and morbidity in the United States of America. *Bulletin of the World Health Organization, 93*(3), 135. doi:10.2471/BLT.14.148627

Amankwaa, L., Records, K., Kenner, C., Roux, G., Stone, S., & Walker, D. (2018). African-American mothers' persistent excessive maternal death rates. *Nursing Outlook, 66*(3), 316–318. doi:10.1016/j.outlook.2018.03.006

American Association of Birth Centers. (2018, November 9). *New government report recommends birth center care* [Press release]. Retrieved from https://www.birthcenters .org/news/426371/New-Government-Report-Recommends-Birth-Center-Care.htm

American Association of Colleges of Nursing. (2010). *Joint statement from the Tri-Council for Nursing on recent registered nurse supply and demand projects.* Retrieved from http://tricouncilfornursing.org/documents/JointStatementRecentRNSupplyDemand Projections.pdf

American College of Obstetricians and Gynecologists. (2013). ACOG committee Opinion No. 554: Reproductive and sexual coercion. *Obstetrics and Gynecology, 121*(2 Pt. 1), 411–415. doi:10.1097/01.AOG.0000426427.79586.3b

Amnesty International. (2011). *Deadly delivery: The maternal health care crisis in the USA: One-year update.* New York, NY: Author. Retrieved from https://cdn2.sph.harvard .edu/wp-content/uploads/sites/32/2017/06/deadlydeliveryoneyear.pdf

Bartlett, L., Weissman, E., Gubin, R., Patton-Molitors, R., & Friberg, I. (2014). The impact and cost of scaling up midwifery and obstetrics in 58 low- and middle-income countries. *PLoS ONE, 9*(6), e98550. doi:10.1371/journal.pone.0098550

Bergevin, Y., Faveau, V., & McKinnon, B. (2015). Towards ending preventable maternal deaths by 2035. *Seminars in Reproductive Medicine, 33*(1), 23–29. doi:10.1055/s-0034-1395275

Bowser, D., & Hill. K. (2010, September 20). *Exploring evidence for disrespect and abuse in facility-based childbirth: Report of a landscape analysis.* Bethesda, MD: USAID-TRAction Project, University Research Corporation, LLC, & Harvard School of Public Health.

Building U.S. Capacity to Review and Prevent Maternal Deaths. (2018). *Report from nine maternal mortality review committees.* Retrieved from http://reviewtoaction.org/ Report_from_Nine_MMRCs

California Maternal Quality Care Collaborative. (2018). Toolkits. Retrieved from https:// www.cmqcc.org/resources-tool-kits/toolkits

CBS News. (2018, July 26). *U.S. "most dangerous" place to give birth in developed world,* USA Today *investigation finds.* Retrieved from https://www.cbsnews.com/news/us-most -dangerous-place-to-give-birth-in-developed-world-usa-today-investigation-finds

Centers for Disease Control and Prevention. (2017a). Pregnancy mortality surveillance system. Retrieved from https://www.cdc.gov/reproductivehealth/maternalinfanthealth/ pmss.html

Centers for Disease Control and Prevention. (2017b). Severe maternal morbidity in the United States. Retrieved from https://www.cdc.gov/reproductivehealth/maternalinfant health/severematernalmorbidity.html

Central Intelligence Agency. (2018, January 1). *World Factbook.* Retrieved from https:// www.cia.gov/library/publications/the-world-factbook/rankorder/2223rank.html

Cheng, T., & Solomon, B. (2014). Translating Life Course Theory to clinical practice to address health disparities. *Maternal and Child Health Journal, 18*(2), 389–395. doi:10.1007/ s10995-013-1279-9

Clark, S., & Belfort, M. (2017). The case for a national maternal mortality review committee. *Obstetrics and Gynecology, 130*(1), 198–202. doi:10.1097/AOG.0000000000002062

Commemorating women's day, Annan calls for prioritizing women's needs. (2003, March 7). *UN News*. Retrieved from https://news.un.org/en/story/2003/03/61252-commemo rating-womens-day-annan-calls-prioritizing-womens-needs

Council on Patient Safety in Women's Health Care. (n.d.). Patient safety bundles. Retrieved from https://safehealthcareforeverywoman.org/patient-safety-bundles

Creanga, A. (2018). Maternal mortality in the United States: A review of contemporary data and their limitations. *Clinical Obstetrics and Gynecology, 61*(2), 296–306. doi:10.1097/GRF.0000000000000362

Creanga, A., Berg, C., Ko, J., Farr, S., Tong, V., Bruce, F., & Callaghan, W. (2014). Maternal mortality and morbidity in the United States: Where are we now? *Journal of Women's Health, 23*(1), 3–9. doi:10.1089/jwh.2013.4617

Dawley, K., & Walsh, L. (2016). Creating a more diverse midwifery workforce in the United States: A historical reflection. *Journal of Midwifery and Women's Health, 61*(5), 578–585. doi:10.1111/jmwh.12489

Fay, K., & Yee, L. (2018). Reproductive coercion and women's health. *Journal of Midwifery and Women's Health, 63*(5), 518–525. doi:10.1111/jmwh.12885

Global Burden of Disease Study Maternal Mortality Collaborators. (2016). Global, regional and national levels of maternal mortality, 1990–2015: A systematic analysis for the Global Burden of Disease Study 2015. *Lancet, 388*(10053), 1775–1812. doi:10.1016/S0140-6736(16)31470-2

Halfon, N., Larson, K., Lu, M., Tullis, E., & Russ, S. (2014). Lifecourse health development: Past, present and future. *Maternal and Child Health Journal, 18*(2), 344–365. doi:10.1007/s10995-013-1346-2

Homer, C., Friberg, I., Bastos Dias, M., ten Hoope-Bender, P., Sandall, J., Speciale, A., & Bartlett, L. (2014). The projected effect of scaling up midwifery. *Lancet, 384*(9948), 1146–1157. doi:10.1016/S0140-6736(14)60790-X

Hutchison, M., Ennis, L., Shaw-Battista, J., Delgado, A., Myers, K., Cragin, L., & Jackson, R. (2011). Great minds don't think alike: Collaborative maternity care at San Francisco General Hospital. *Obstetrics & Gynecology, 118*(3), 678–682. doi:10.1097/AOG.0b013e3182297d2d

Institute of Medicine and the Robert Wood Johnson Foundation. (2010). *The future of nursing: Leading change, advancing health*. Washington, DC: National Academies Press. Retrieved from http://www.nationalacademies.org/hmd/Reports/2010/The-Future-of-Nursing-Leading-Change-Advancing-Health.aspx

Kennedy, H., Cheyney, M., Dahlen, H., Downe, S., Foureur, M., Homer, C., . . . Renfrew, M. (2018). Asking different questions: A call to action for research to improve the quality of care for every woman, every child. *Birth, 45*(3), 222–231. doi:10.1111/birt.12361

Kennedy, H., & Waldman, R. (Eds.). (2012). Collaborative practice in obstetrics and gynecology [Special issue]. *Obstetrics and Gynecology Clinics of North America, 39*(3), 323–452.

Kozhimannil, K., Casey, M., Hung, P., Han, X., Prasad, S., & Moscovice, I. (2015). The rural obstetric workforce in US hospitals: Challenges and opportunities. *Journal of Rural Health, 31*(4), 365–372. doi:10.1111/jrh.12112

MacDorman, M., & Declercq, E. (2018). The failure of the United States maternal mortality reporting and its impact on women's lives. *Birth, 45,* 105–108. doi:10.1111/birt .12333

Mischler, A. E. (2017). Paradise is at her feet. Retrieved from https://muslimvillage.com/ 2017/01/05/10093/paradise-at-the-feet-of-your-mother

Mitchell, P., Wynia, R., Golden, R., McNellis B., Okun, S., Webb, C., . . . Von Kohorn, I. (2012). *Core principles & values of effective team-based health care [Discussion paper].* Washington, DC: Institute of Medicine. Retrieved from https://nam.edu/wp-content/ uploads/2015/06/VSRT-Team-Based-Care-Principles-Values.pdf

Neerland, C. (2018). Maternal confidence for physiologic childbirth: A concept analysis. *Journal of Midwifery and Women's Health, 63*(4), 425–435. doi:10.1111/jmwh.12719

Patient Protection and Affordable Care Act, 42 U.S.C. § 18001 et seq. (2010).

Peck, E. (2018, May 27). Everyone is missing a key reason the U.S. birth rate is declining. *Huffington Post.* Retrieved from https://www.huffingtonpost.com/entry/key-reason -birth-rate-declining_us_5b0725cfe4b0568a88097feb

Shekelle, P. G., Wachter, R. M., Pronovost, P. J., Schoelles, K., McDonald, K. M., Dy, S. M., . . . Winters, B. D. (2013). *Making health care safer II: An updated critical analysis of the evidence for patient safety practices* (AHRQ Publication No. 13-E001-EF). Rockville, MD: Agency for Healthcare Research and Quality. Retrieved from http://www.ahrq .gov/research/findings/evidence-based-reports/ptsafetyuptp.html

Smith, V., Gifford, K., Ellis, E., Edwards, B., Rudowitz, R., Hinton, E., . . . Valentine, A. (2017) *Implementing coverage and payment initiatives: Results from a 50-state Medicaid budget survey for state fiscal years 2016 and 2017.* Retrieved from https://www .kff.org/medicaid/report/implementing-coverage-and-payment-initiatives-results -from-a-50-state-medicaid-budget-survey-for-state-fiscal-years-2016-and-2017

St. Pierre, A., Zaharatos, J., Goodman, D., & Callaghan, W. (2018). Challenges and opportunities in identifying, reviewing, and preventing maternal deaths. *Obstetrics and Gynecology, 131*(1), 138–142. doi:10.1097/AOG.0000000000002417

Task Force on Collaborative Practice. (2016). *Collaboration in practice: Implementing team-based care.* Washington, DC: American College of Obstetricians and Gynecologists.

Waldman, R., Kennedy, H., & Kendig, S. (2012). Collaboration in maternity care: Possibilities and challenges. *Obstetrics and Gynecology Clinics of North America, 39*(3), 435–444. doi:10.1016/j.ogc.2012.05.011

The White Ribbon Alliance. (2012). *Respectful maternity care: The universal rights of childbearing women.* Retrieved from http://www.who.int/woman_child_accountability/ ierg/reports/2012_01S_Respectful_Maternity_Care_Charter_The_Universal_Rights _of_Childbearing_Women.pdf

Williams, D. (2016). How racism makes us sick. *TED Talk*. Retrieved from https://www
.ted.com/talks/david_r_williams_how_racism_makes_us_sick?utm_source=
tedcomshare&utm_medium=email&utm_campaign=tedspread

Woolf, S., & Aron, L. (Eds.). (2013). *U.S. health in international perspective: Shorter lives,
poorer health*. Washington, DC: National Academies Press.

AFTERWORD

As well described in this book, the maternal mortality and morbidity crisis in America is unprecedented. As we continue to spend more and more on maternity care, our outcomes continue to decline. Of great concern is the fact that research is telling us that more than half of the deaths are preventable. There are many reasons for this trend and many evidence-based strategies being proposed and implemented that show some promise of improving the problem. A major focus is the care provided within the healthcare system. Studies show us that difficulty accessing care, lack of evidence-based and standardized care, especially within hospitals, and poor communication between providers and patients all contribute to the poor outcomes. There are promising strategies being implemented in some hospitals in the form of standardized bundles to decrease the cesarean section rate and manage severe illness and obstetrical emergencies (Council on Patient Safety in Women's Health Care, n.d.). While these are important and much needed, we need to take a giant step backward and look at the big picture if we are going to make significant improvements. That is the strength of this book.

Care for women, either in labor or with a health crisis, cannot start upon admission to the hospital. We have to address the many issues that lead to that point. Women need access to culturally competent healthcare at every junction, including when trying to avoid pregnancy, when preparing for a pregnancy, during pregnancy, during the postpartum period, and between pregnancies. Rising maternal mortality is a complex issue and contributing factors extend beyond medical complications. These include financial and bureaucratic issues, geographical accessibility, lack of culturally competent care, and racism. Care must include healthcare providers who have the education, time, and desire to listen, reflect, teach, and brainstorm with women about their situations, their options for care, and strategies to improve their health. This is the reason that to improve the health of women, we need teams of healthcare providers, including at least midwives, nurses, obstetricians, public health nurses, and community health workers (CHWs). Our current healthcare system in the United States relies primarily on obstetricians to provide care during pregnancy. This is not sustainable. The American College of Obstetricians and Gynecologists (ACOG) predicts an increasing shortage of obstetricians (Rayburn, 2017). Further, there is evidence that women who receive care in midwife-led models are less likely to experience intervention and more likely to be satisfied with their care (Sandall, Soltani, Gates, Shennan, & Devane, 2016). Incorporating midwives can lead to increased accessibility of care. CHWs work as part of the maternity team to meet in women's homes to assess, educate, and connect families with needed services. Including CHWs in the plan has shown to improve access to care and health outcomes (Association of State and Territorial Health Officials [ASTHO], 2017). The greatest percentage of maternal mortality occurs after the birth. Reinstituting public health nurse visits in the postpartum period could help identify serious issues such as difficulties with lactation, ongoing preeclampsia, and postpartum depression. The bottom line is that it will take a team approach to improve maternal mortality and morbidity. We must engage in the community and the family with care models that involve different types of providers in teams. Doing what we have always done is not going to improve the situation.

It is important that we understand our role in advocating for high-quality and accessible healthcare. Accessibility begins with the ability to afford healthcare. We must consistently remind our legislators of this fact. We must lobby for adequate insurance coverage for *all* women. Next, we need funding for studies that demonstrate how to improve health outcomes. Legislation that funds programs such as maternal mortality review committees and recognition of maternity shortage areas is critical to the identification of the root causes and the development and funding of strategies to improve health. As healthcare providers, we need to understand that we are the ones who can help legislators understand the importance of such programs. Most legislators are not steeped in the issues of the healthcare system and need our help in understanding why these issues are important.

In the preceding pages, readers were able to take a deeper look at the issues women are facing in the United States in attaining adequate care during their childbearing years. The importance of examining the social determinants of health in relation to maternal mortality and morbidity is critical as we continue to seek solutions.

Susan E. Stone, DNSc, RN, CNM, FACNM, FAAN
President, American College of Nurse-Midwives
President, Frontier Nursing University
Lexington, Kentucky

REFERENCES

Association of State and Territorial Health Officials. (2017). *Utilizing community health workers to improve access to care for maternal and child populations: Four state approaches* [Issue brief]. Retrieved from http://www.astho.org/Maternal-and-Child-Health/AIM-Access-CHW-Issue-Brief

Council on Patient Safety in Women's Health Care. (2018). Patient safety bundles. Retrieved from https://safehealthcareforeverywoman.org/patient-safety-bundles

Rayburn, W. (2017). *The obstetrician gynecologist workforce in the US: Facts, figures, and implications*. Washington, DC: American Congress of Obstetricians and Gynecologists.

Sandall, J., Soltani, H., Gates S., Shennan, A., & Devane, D. (2016). Midwife-led continuity models versus other models of care for childbearing women. *Cochrane Database of Systematic Reviews, 2016*(4), CD004667. doi:10.1002/14651858.CD004667.pub5

APPENDIX A

Selected Advocacy Resources With Focus on Maternal Health

ORGANIZATION	DESCRIPTION	WEBSITE
American Academy of Family Physicians	Advocating for legislation to reduce maternal mortality in the United States	https://www.aafp.org/home.html
American Academy of Nursing	Advancing health policy and practice in nursing	http://www.aannet.org/home
American Association of Nurse-Practitioners	Advocating for NP voice pertaining to all health policy matters and excellence in patient care, including maternal health	https://www.aanp.org
American College of Nurse-Midwives	Advocating for midwifery practice and high-quality, high-value care for women and their babies	http://www.midwife.org
American College of Obstetricians and Gynecologists	Advocating to ensure lawmakers support OB/GYN patients and practices and supporting policies to protect women and the specialty	https://www.acog.org
American Nurses Association	Advocating for policies aimed to improve healthcare for all, including pregnant women	https://www.nursingworld.org
American Public Health Association	Working with key decision makers to shape public policy to address today's ongoing public health concerns and safe motherhood in the United States	https://www.apha.org

(continued)

APPENDIX A (*continued*)

ORGANIZATION	DESCRIPTION	WEBSITE
Amnesty International	Campaigning for a world where human rights are enjoyed by all, including mothers everywhere	https://www.amnesty.org/en
Association of Maternal & Child Health Programs	Advocating for state public health leaders and others working to improve the health of women	http://www.amchp.org/Pages/default.aspx
Association of Women's Health, Obstetric and Neonatal Nurses (AWHONN)	Supporting nurses caring for women, newborns, and their families through research, education, and advocacy	https://www.awhonn.org
Black Mamas Matter Alliance	A Black women–led cross-sectoral alliance, focusing on advocacy, research, building power, and shifting culture for Black maternal health, rights, and justice	https://blackmamasmatter.org
CDC National Partnership to Eliminate Preventable Maternal Deaths	Promoting the maternal mortality review process as the best way to understand why maternal mortality in the United States is increasing, and identify interventions to prevent maternal deaths	https://www.cdcfoundation.org/building-us-capacity-review-and-prevent-maternal-deaths
Childbirth Connection	Developing and advancing critical components of the maternity care system, including promoting evidence-based maternity care through policy and quality initiatives	http://www.childbirthconnection.org
Choices in Childbirth Centre for Social Innovation	Providing expectant parents with information and education so they can experience the birth they choose	http://choicesinchildbirth.org
Collaborative for Alcohol-Free Pregnancy	Promoting prevention of fetal alcohol spectrum disorders (FASDs) and alcohol-exposed pregnancies	https://www.cdc.gov/ncbddd/fasd/alcohol-use.html
Every Mother Counts	Working to make pregnancy and childbirth safe for every mother, everywhere, by educating the public about maternal health and investing in programs to improve access to essential maternity care	http://www.everymothercounts.org

(*continued*)

APPENDIX A (*continued*)

ORGANIZATION	DESCRIPTION	WEBSITE
Full Circle Doula	Supporting birth with continuous emotional, physical, and informational support during labor, birth, and the immediate postpartum period	www.fullcircledoulagroup.com
International Cesarean Awareness Network (ICAN)	Improving maternal–child health by reducing preventable cesareans through education, supporting cesarean recovery, and advocating for vaginal birth after cesarean (VBAC)	http://www.ican-online.org
International Childbirth Education Association (ICEA)	Supporting educators and healthcare professionals toward family-centered maternity and newborn care	https://icea.org
Lamaze International	Offering accredited childbirth education certification to prepare parents to make informed decisions	https://www.lamaze.org
March for Moms	Building coalition sharing to improve the well-being of mothers in the United States	http://www.marchformoms.org
Merck for Mothers	Improving the health and well-being of mothers before, during, and after pregnancy and childbirth	http://merckformothers.com
March of Dimes	Supporting legislation to discover the causes of maternal mortality and empower states to avert preventable deaths	https://www.marchofdimes.org
Midwives Alliance of North America	Unifying and strengthening the midwifery profession to improve the quality of maternal healthcare	https://mana.org
Preeclampsia Foundation	Supporting efforts to reduce maternal and infant illness and death due to preeclampsia, HELLP syndrome, and other hypertensive disorders of pregnancy	https://www.preeclampsia.org

(continued)

APPENDIX A (*continued*)

ORGANIZATION	DESCRIPTION	WEBSITE
Sister Song	Building a network of individuals and organizations to improve institutional policies and systems that impact the reproductive lives of marginalized communities	https://www.sistersong.net
Society for Maternal–Fetal Medicine: Health Policy/Advocacy Committee	Interacting with members of Congress, their staffs, and key federal agency officials to advocate for maternal health	https://www.smfm.org
Transforming Maternity Care	Advocating for a high-quality, high-value maternity care system and equitable care	https://transform.childbirthconnection.org
White Ribbon Alliance (WRA)	Advocating for global movement for maternal care and prevention of maternal mortality	https://www.whiteribbonalliance.org

CDC, Centers for Disease Control and Prevention; HELLP, hemolysis, elevated liver enzymes, low platelet count; NP, nurse practitioner.

APPENDIX B

The Safe Motherhood Quilt Project

Memorials Honor Those Who Have Died

Memorials are created so we never forget the reasons for the tragic loss of human lives.

Memorials are created so those who died did not die in vain.

Memorials spur us to confront the cause and fight for change so that lives will be saved.

—Suzan Ulrich, DrPH, RN, CNM, FACNM

The Safe Motherhood Quilt Project: Remember the Mothers was created by Ina May Gaskin, a midwifery leader and birth advocate, to call attention to the rising number of mothers dying from pregnancy-related causes as well as the underreporting of these deaths. The quilt includes a memorial square designed to remember each mother who died since 1982. The Safe Motherhood Quilt has been displayed in many places, including the state capitals, the Centers for Disease Control and Prevention, and the United States Capitol, to call attention

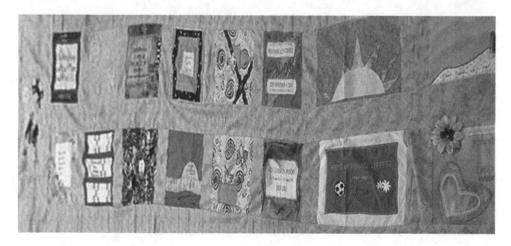

SOURCE: Reproduced with permission from the Bellies to Babies Foundation.

to this tragic loss of mothers. The goal is to promote accurate identification of maternal deaths and analyze root causes that result in recommendations to improve maternity care.

The Safe Motherhood Quilt Project: Remember the Mothers is now being cared for by Bellies to Babies Foundation, a 501c3 nonprofit agency providing education and support to improve childbirth.

RESOURCES

http://rememberthemothers.org

https://www.facebook.com/BelliestoBabiesEvents

https://twitter.com/btobfoundation_

INDEX

Printed in the United States
by Bookmasters

Printed in the United States
By Bookmasters